NOURISH

mind, body & soul

Amber Rose grew up in New Zealand, surrounded by heritage fruit and vegetables in her mother's renowned organic permaculture garden. She is a food stylist and regularly cooks for clients in their homes (including Gwyneth Paltrow and Kate Hudson). In her cooking and baking, Amber focuses on produce-led, traditional diets and nutrient-dense foods and takes her inspiration from the seasons. Her first book was the best-selling *Love Bake Nourish*, translated into five languages.

Sadie Frost lives in London with her four children. Apart from her roles within Fashion with Floozie and Iris and Edie by Frostfrench and her career as an actress, Sadie is currently involved with her film company Blonde to Black Pictures, which has just completed two feature films, with many more to come. Alongside this, Sadie has being doing an MA with Raindance and Staffordshire University in Film Studies. She has always had a keen interest in health and fitness and has studied yoga, meditation and nutrition for nearly 20 years. She recognises that these things enable her to try to achieve the perfect balance to live calmly and to have a certain quality of peace of mind.

Holly Davidson grew up in the English countryside, beginning an active lifestyle from an early age. An established actor in film and television, she performed in dramatic and comedic roles for over ten years. Holly currently practices as a Level 3 personal trainer and fitness coach. Her numerous clients include celebrities Florence Welsh, Nick Grimshaw and Sienna Guillory. Renowned for her enthusiasm to motivate people, Holly is qualified in a range of techniques, such as kick-boxing, Pilates, kettle bells, TRX and post-natal exercises, and advises on nutrition and lifestyle changes. She lives and works in London.

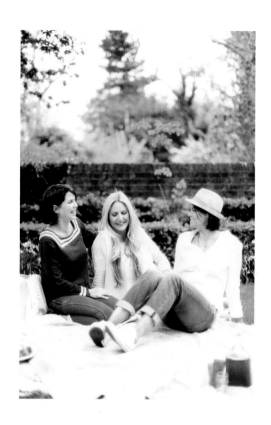

Amber
To my amazing and inspiring son and to all the beautiful, strong
women in my life, and to all the single parents out there –
you are all super heroes.

Sadie
To Fin, Raff, Iris and Rudy, my little babies. And to my mother,
Mary Davidson, and grandmother, Betty Nolan, for being the most
nourishing women I've met.

Holly
To my wonderful mum and dad. Thank you for always believing in
me. I couldn't have chosen better.

NOURISH

Mind, body & soul

Amber Rose, Sadie Frost & Holly Davidson

Photography by David Loftus

Kyle Books

First published in Great Britain in 2014 by Kyle Books,
an imprint of Kyle Cathie Limited,
192-198 Vauxhall Bridge Road,
London SW1V 1DX

general.enquiries@kylebooks.com
www.kylebooks.com

10 9 8 7 6 5 4 3 2 1
ISBN 978085783 2511

A CIP catalogue record for this title is available from the
British Library.

The information and advice contained in this book are
intended as a general guide. Neither the authors nor the
publishers can be held responsible for claims arising from
the inappropriate use of any remedy or exercise regime.
Do not attempt self-diagnosis or self-treatment for serious
or long-term conditions before consulting a medical
professional or qualified practitioner. Do not begin any
exercise programme or undertake any self-treatment
while taking other prescribed drugs or receiving therpay
without first seeking professional guidance. Always seek
medical advice if any symptoms persist.

Text © Amber Rose, Sadie Frost & Holly Davidson 2014

Photographs © David Loftus 2014
Design © Kyle Books 2014

Author coordinator: Amber Rose
Copy editor: Stephanie Evans
Editorial assistant: Tara O'Sullivan
Proofreader: Catherine Ward
Design: BuroCreative
Photographer: David Loftus
Food & props styling: Amber Rose
Stylist: Fabiola De Freitas
Production: Gemma John & Nic Jones
Colour reproduction: ALTA London
Printed and bound in China by C&C Offset
Printing Co., Ltd

CONTENTS

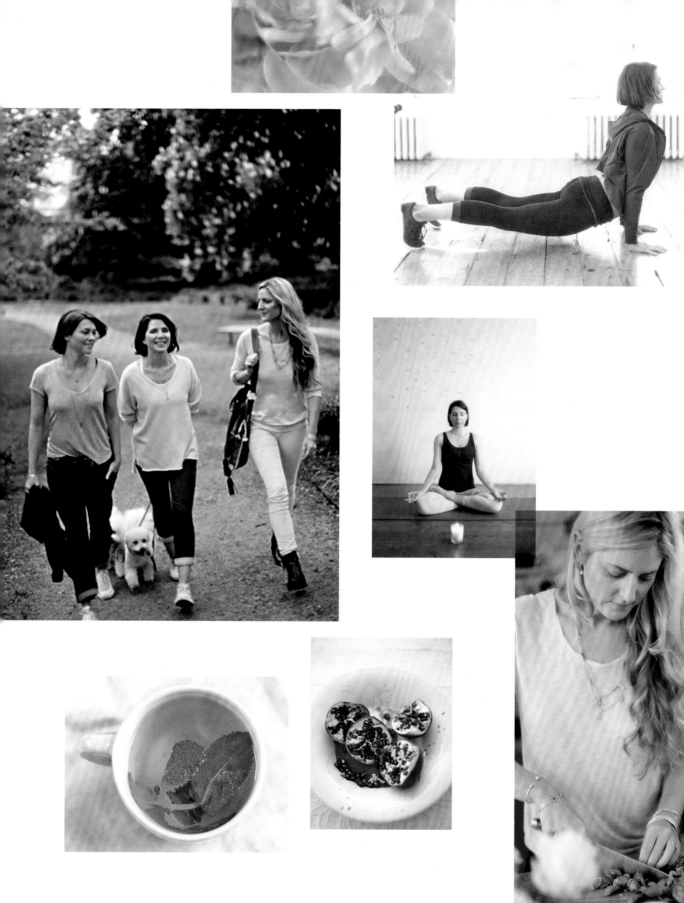

INTRODUCTION

This is a book that covers health and nourishment for the mind, body and soul.

We are three women, we are three friends, we are three people passionate about food, wellbeing and exercise. In one way or another we have all been on a journey that has involved health issues and struggles with the pressures of life. In this book we share with you the tips, tricks, solutions and answers that we have learned along the way to get our bodies back in shape, to get our health back on track after illness, to still our minds amongst the stresses of family and life, or just to maintain a positive and happy outlook and, above all, to have fun.

For each of us, this book is about sharing information, amongst women, families and generations. It's about wisdom and nourishment. It's about community and coming together to support each other to lead the happiest and best lives we can, to feel that we have a few tricks up our sleeves and tools in our tool box - so that even when obstacles block our path, we have the knowledge and support to get over them, around them or under them and back on track.

The book is arranged into three major sections: food, mind and body, with Holly Davidson bringing you amazing exercise routines and plans to strengthen and inspire, to get you motivated or to push you through to the next level to up your game. Holly's enthusiasm is infectious and inspiring and her exercise programmes are easy to follow with fantastic results.

In Sadie Frost's section you will find her sharing her gorgeous home beauty recipes and remedies to soothe tired skin, to bring a shine back to your hair or simply to pamper yourself after a gruelling week. Sadie also shares her knowledge of meditation, yoga and mindfulness to encourage peace of mind and contentment. Such useful tools for anyone to have…

Amber Rose shares the recipes that she uses on a daily basis to support health and happiness. They are seasonal, nutrient-dense recipes that can be cooked to nourish the body, strengthen the immune system and heal a stressed digestive system. They are the recipes that she cooks for family and friends during a busy week, a lazy weekend breakfast or a big celebration; whatever the occasion, there is always a way to stay healthy and keep it delicious.

In this book we hope that you find knowledge, support and nourishment that will help you on your journey, as it has ours. Enjoy.

Love,
Amber, Sadie & Holly x

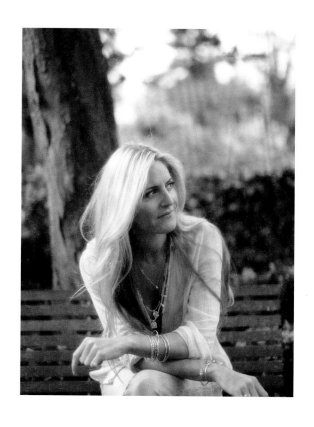
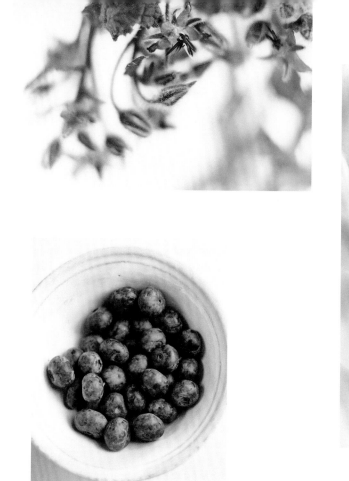
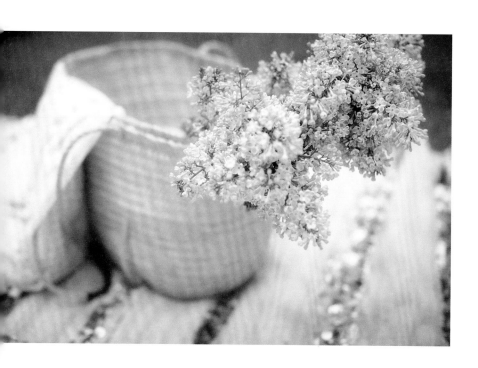
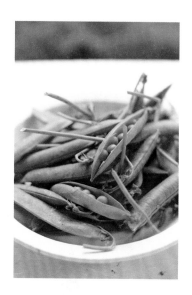

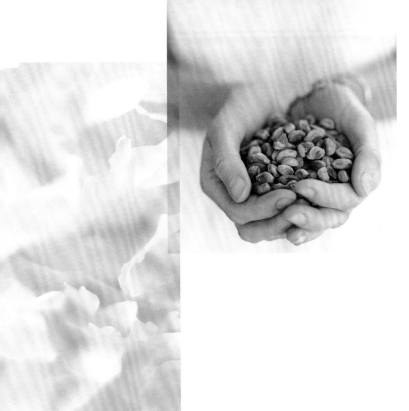

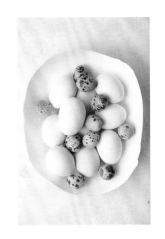

SUPER-FOOD

Amber

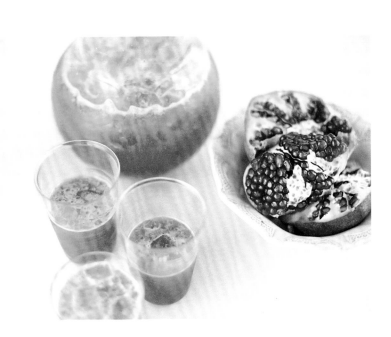

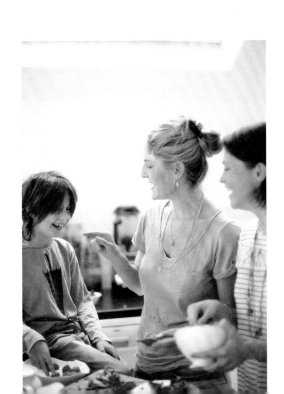

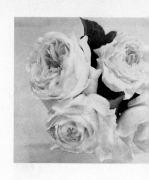

I enjoyed a free-range childhood, spending my days eating and cooking from my mother's garden, picking wild flowers and foraging for wild fruits and berries and other delights. I would happily forsake a clean dress if it meant I could just reach that ripest, juiciest and most delicious blackberry at the very top of the prickliest and highest cane. I have always loved eating but have also loved the process of gathering, collecting and preparing the food. The ingredients we gather and cook are what sustain us and those we love.

Food is such an integral part of lives, families and greater communities. It can define who we are, how we relate to one another and how we feel about ourselves. I love the way food can bring people together. Community has always been a big thing for me. I am connected to those around me, the people I love, through expression, and one of the ways I express myself is through food. Food can be warming, earthy and robust – exactly what we need for those cold winter months when days are short and we need comfort and sustenance of the highest order – or it can be light, delicate and gentle, or restorative, or cleansing, for the warmer lighter spring and summer months. The way we eat greatly determines how we feel about ourselves. It's easy to forget that sometimes. Food is medicine

Food is such an integral part of lives, families and greater communities. It can define who we are, how we relate to one another and how we feel about ourselves.

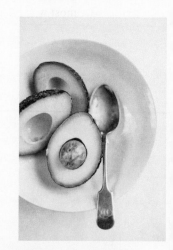

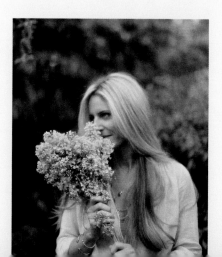

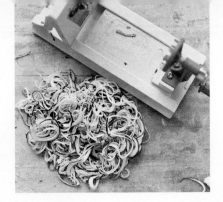

and medicine is food. The idea that we can adapt what and how we eat to alter how we feel within ourselves is empowering. My style of cooking and baking is produce led and based on traditional diets with nutrient-dense foods, healthy fats and heritage produce. This is how my mother cooked for me, and how I choose to cook for my family and those I love. Making nourishing meals is serious business but that doesn't mean it can't also be playful, easy to prepare and above all a pleasure to eat and share with those around you.

I have never had any formal training. I am a self-taught cook, but I have had a passion and a love for good food passed down to me by a mother who has one of the most wonderful gardens in New Zealand, filled with over 800 varieties of heritage fruit and vegetables, and a father who was a chef. Our pantry was my mother's garden, an open-air larder, if you like. As a little girl I would find things in my mother's veg patch to harvest and cook. Over the years, that hasn't really changed much – there's a very seasonal and flexible approach to creating my menus; my style of cooking is very simple, with lots of fresh herbs thrown in for good measure. And what I feed my son is what I eat myself. He is a great eater and I feel that is partly because I choose to eat with him and we always share

that moment of the day together. From an early age he would pick bits of salad off my plate and try new things because he saw me enjoying it he thought he would give it a go. Mealtimes should be shared and always a pleasure. This is how children grow to love and understand food.

The inspiration for me to write this book has been based on my feelings about families, community, friends, sharing, loving, learning and growing. I find it quite wonderful that three friends can come together to share what they have learnt from different walks of life to support one another as well as women everywhere so that we can all support ourselves and our families.

I am a single parent and without my community of friends around me I wouldn't be where I am today. For me, this book is about sharing with you what I have learnt along the way – from that free-range childhood through to supporting women through childbirth as a doula, and from being a mum myself to being a friend and someone who loves to share my knowledge and support with anyone who wants it.

Lots of love,
Amber x

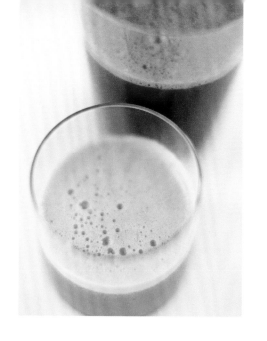

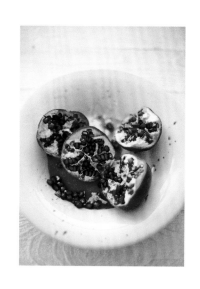

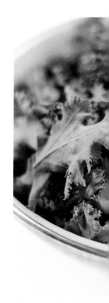

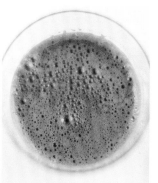

SMOOTHIES

&

JUICES

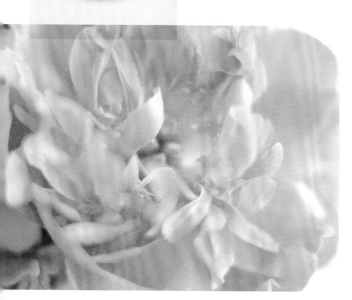

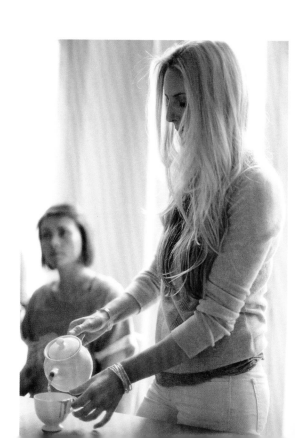

This is a chapter that includes juices, smoothies, delicious fruity waters, hot drinks and my favourite hot chocolate of all time – you just won't believe is so good and also so good for you! Juices and smoothies are a great way to start the morning.

I often have a juice or a smoothie for breakfast during the week when I am busy and rushing around. I find a big breakfast doesn't always work for me during the week. Juices and smoothies are really cleansing and nourishing and they are a great way of getting all the nutrients and energy that you need for your morning without the heavy feeling a big breakfast can give you if you're busy and up early. Don't get me wrong, though, I love big breakfasts! I just usually save them for the weekend and turn them into a leisurely affair. I spent my childhood wandering through my mother's gardens, picking herbs and flowers for tea and always choose a fresh herb tea over a dried one.

Fresh herb tea is so so easy to make and if you have herbs in your garden or even some dried herbs in jars you can make up combos that suit what you feel like. I love adding lemon or lime to pots of fresh herb tea. Fresh tea has a lot more going for it than anything you will get from a bag, and it's just as quick and easy. Of course, there are moments when nothing but a perfectly brewed cup of Earl Grey tea will do, and on those occasions I love nothing more than a pot with some raw milk or my favourite homemade almond milk, sweetened with a touch of honey – perfection ! The two biggest benefits to making your own juices and smoothies are that 1)they taste amazing, much better than anything you can buy in a bottle; and 2) because they are freshly made from whole fruit and not packaged, they have not been pasteurised, as pretty much all juices and smoothies you will find on a supermarket shelf have been. The process of pasteurisation kills off all the beneficial enzymes, which are what help you to digest any of the goodness in the fruit or veg. When you buy bottled juices and smoothies, you are pretty much just drinking sugar, unless they are cold pressed, unpasteurised and very fresh.

Another good thing to remember is that by adding kefir or full fat coconut milk to smoothies, you are adding the 'good fats' that make all the micro nutrients bio-available. To get around this when juicing, I always add some good seed or nut oils to my fresh juices, or even some cod liver oil – there are some great brands out there that don't have a fishy taste but do provide you with your essential fatty acids. So there you have it, a few great reasons why making your own drinks is not only super delicious but also nourishing and rewarding for your body.

A DELICIOUS GREEN SMOOTHIE

This is my most favourite smoothie, it's simply the goodness of the greens. Perfection.

1 small banana, peeled, sliced and frozen ahead of time
Handful of spinach or kale, washed and drained
1 scoop of your favourite powdered super greens
1 teaspoon raw coconut oil
1 teaspoon either fish oils or your favourite omega oil
1 teaspoon raw honey
300 ml filtered water or almond milk or coconut water

Place all the ingredients in a blender and blitz until completely smooth.

SUPER RED BERRY & KEFIR SMOOTHIE

Milk kefir is so full of probiotics and enzymes and it has a wonderful slightly sour tangy taste, which balances with the berries perfectly. Kefir helps with digestion and supports the immune system. This is great smoothie for both kids and adults.

250ml milk kefir
1 tablespoon raw honey
1 teaspoon raw coconut oil
½ large banana, previously frozen, sliced
Handful of any frozen red berries (strawberries, raspberries, redcurrants)
1 heaped tablespoon goji berries, soaked overnight in filtered water and drained

Put everything into a blender and blitz for 2 minutes or until completely smooth.

Drink and enjoy.

BLACKBERRY, ROSE & RAW CHOCOLATE SMOOTHIE

It's great for kids and adults. You may want to leave the rosewater out for the kids, it's quite a grown up flavor, but a delightful one for those who love it, ie me!

1 large banana, peeled
a large handful of frozen blackberries, or blackcurrants or a mix (must be frozen)
1 heaped teaspoon raw coconut oil
1 teaspoon raw honey
1 teaspoon rosewater
2 teaspoons raw cacao powder
½ teaspoon cacao nibs (optional)
250ml almond milk

Place all of your prepared ingredients into a blender and blitz for 2 minutes or until completely smooth.

Pour into a glass and sprinkle with the cacao nibs.

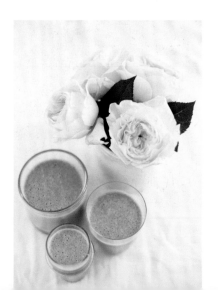

Red berries are full of antioxidants.

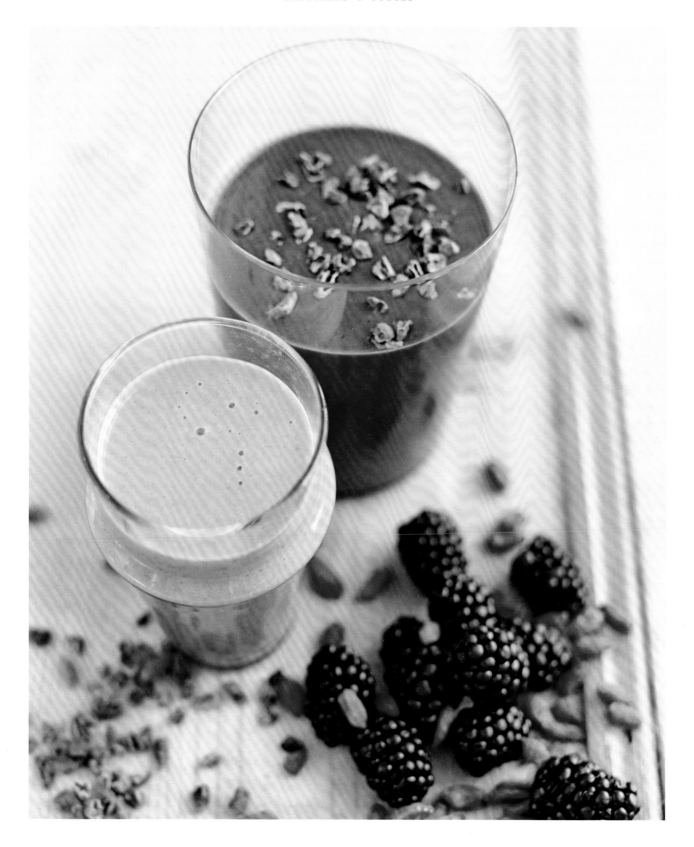

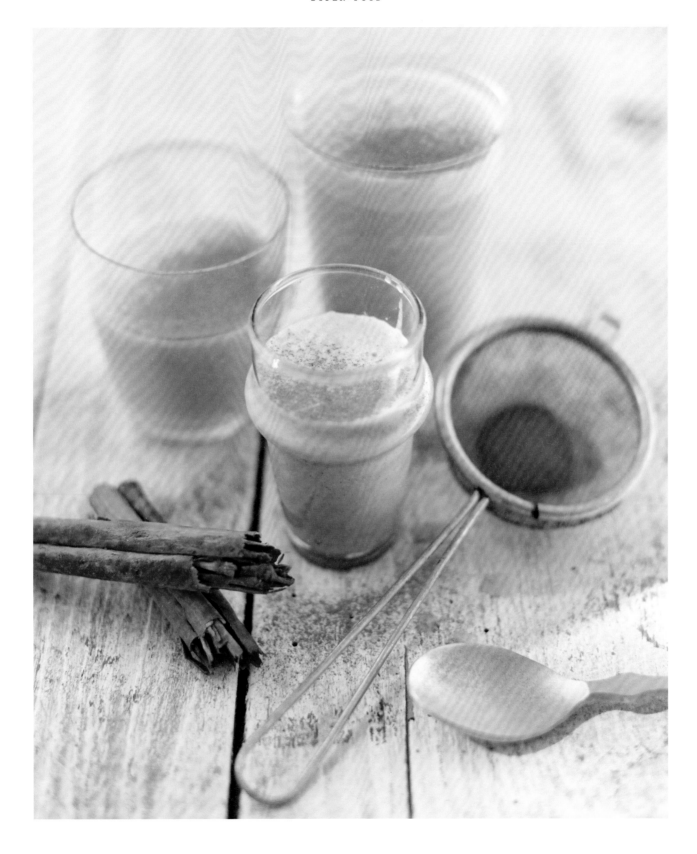

BANANA & ALMOND SMOOTHIE

with Cinnamon

This is a wonderful smoothie. I usually have a few frozen bananas knocking about in my freezer and cinnamon is a staple in the pantry so it's easy to rustle up and is one that both adults and kids love. Cinnamon is great for curbing sweet cravings and pairs beautifully with the banana.

1 large banana, previously frozen, sliced
300ml fresh almond milk
1 hearty teaspoon almond butter
1 teaspoon raw coconut oil
¼ teaspoon cinnamon
½ teaspoon raw honey

Toppings to serve
Handful of soaked raw almonds,
  drained and roughly chopped (optional)
A dusting of cinnamon

Blitz all the ingredients in a blender until smooth. Pour into a glass and sprinkle with a little extra cinnamon and some chopped nuts if you like.

MEAN GREEN MORNING SMOOTHIE

with Extra Protein

Protein is an important part of your diet and nuts are a really good source, especially for vegetarians and vegans.

1 small handful of soaked raw almonds or cashews
1 tablespoon almond nut butter
2 medjool dates, pitted
4 kale leaves, stalks removed, washed and chopped
1 teaspoon your favourite powdered super greens
250ml kefir, or unsweetened almond milk
1 large handful of ice cubes

Simply place everything into a blender and blitz for 2 minutes, or until completely smooth. For a thinner consistency, add a little more kefir, almond milk or water and blitz again.

BEET KVASS

Beet Kvass is an amazing health tonic, it has powerful medicinal qualities and it acts as a digestive aid. Beets are packed full of nutrients. One small glass in the morning and night is an excellent blood tonic; it promotes regularity, aids digestion, alkalizes the blood, cleanses the liver and is a good treatment for kidney stones and other ailments. It's an inexpensive health tonic that is made from fermented beets. It has a wonderful savoury, earthy, slightly sour and tangy flavor. Before I tried this for the first time I wasn't expecting to like it, but I love beets and it quickly grew on me and now I love it and would even go so far as to say I crave it.

Makes 1 large 2.5l jar
2–4 beets, depending on size
¼ cup 50ml whey (see notes below on how to make whey)
1 tablespoon sea salt or Himalayan salt (not table salt)
filtered water (NOT tap water: the chlorine will prevent fermentation)
A large 2.5l glass jar, sterilised (this can be done in the dishwasher)

Wash and peel beets and chop them into small cubes roughly 2cm across.

Place the beets in the bottom of your glass jar. Add the whey and salt, then fill the jar with filtered water. Cover with a tea towel or cheese cloth and leave on the counter for two days to ferment. Transfer the whole jar, with a tightly fitted lid, to the fridge.

To drink, simply ladle off a small amount – roughly 80ml – morning and night. When the liquid is finished you can eat the beets at the bottom if you like; these are now what you call lacto fermented veg. The beet kvass will last well in the fridge for several months, by which time you will most likely have polished it off.

*to make whey, simply place about 350ml of natural unsweetened yoghurt (not Greek yoghurt) in a cheesecloth, tie it up and hang it over a bowl. I do this in my sink and tie the cheesecloth to the tap with a piece of string. The thin white liquid that starts to drip from the bottom is whey. By adding whey to the beet kvass mix you will stop any unfriendly bacteria from growing. The leftover natural yoghurt is now like Greek yoghurt, which is delicious.

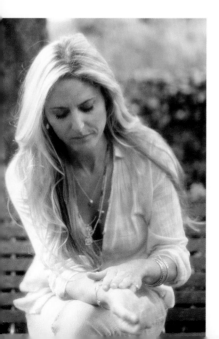

It has powerful medicinal qualities and acts as a digestive aid.

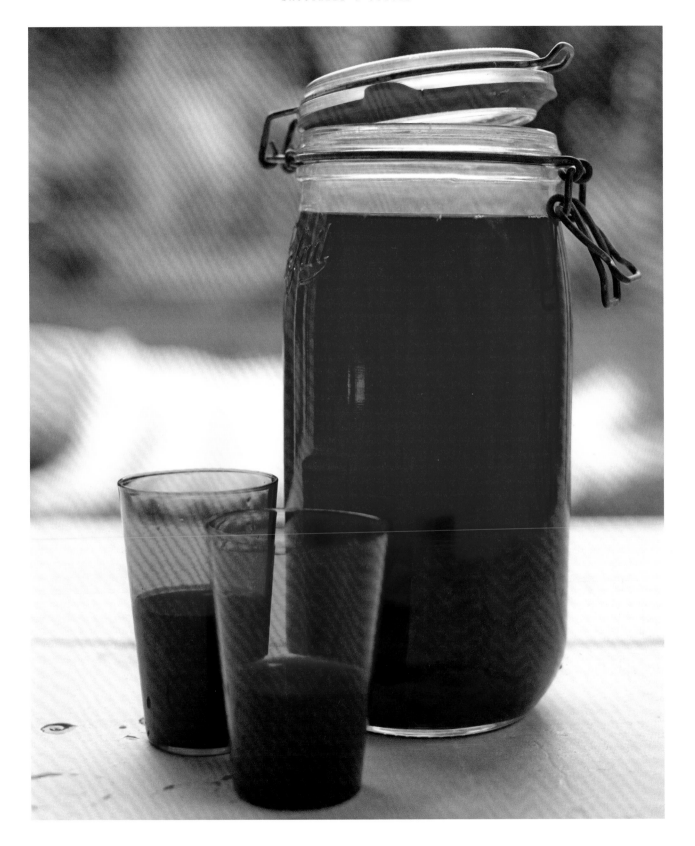

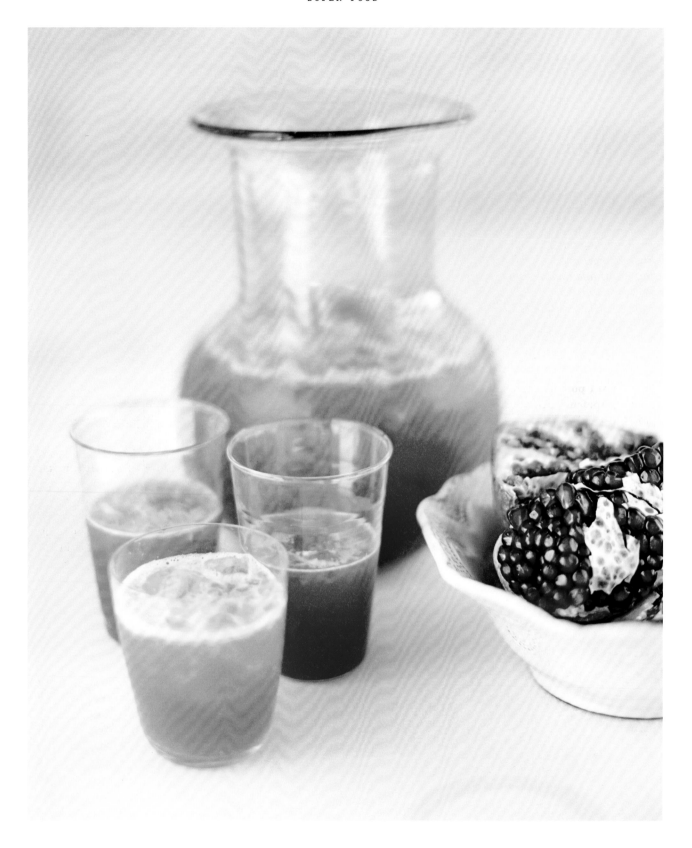

BLOOD ORANGE, POMEGRANATE & GRAPEFRUIT JUICE

This beautifully coloured drink is packed full of anthocyanins. These are powerful antioxidants come from the intense colour of the blood oranges and the pinks in the grapefruits and the dark reds of the pomegranate. It's a special treat when the blood oranges are in season.

4 blood oranges, peeled
  and quartered
Seeds from 1 pomegranate
½ pink grapefruit, peeled
  and halved
¼ lemon, peeled

Wash and prepare your fruit, put through the juicer and drink immediately.

GREEN JUICE

This green juice is nourishing, cleansing and delicious. The mint really lifts the flavour and giving it a refreshing zing.

1 green apple
½ cucumber
½ fennel bulb
Handful of kale
1 kiwi fruit, peeled
3 sprigs of mint
3 stems of parsley
¼ peeled lemon
Small piece of ginger, peeled

Wash all the ingredients, put everything through a juicer and drink immediately.

ABC
with Ginger & Turmeric

I love having a juice before 10am when the liver is in full cleanse mode. Juicing first thing helps your system to cleanse and refresh and start fully loaded with enzymes and immune supporting goodness. If you can't find fresh turmeric, use a pinch of turmeric powder.

1 apple
1 medium beetroot
6 carrots
Small piece of ginger, peeled
Small piece of fresh turmeric,
  peeled
¼ lemon, peeled
1 teaspoon your favourite omega
  or fish oils
freshly cracked black pepper

Wash all the fruit and veg and put thru the juicer. Add the oils and a twist of black pepper. Drink immediately.

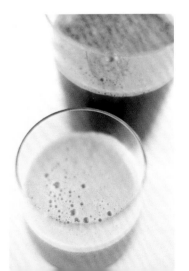

GINGER TEA

with honey

This is the simplest of teas, but so good and so easy. It's alkalising and perfect throughout the day.

A few slices of fresh root ginger, peeled
1 teaspoon raw honey

Boil your kettle, fill your tea cup or mug, gently place the slices of ginger into the boiling water and then allow to sit for a minute or two, before adding the honey.

ALKALISING CIDER VINEGAR TEA *with Raw Honey*

This is a great tea to start the day with, it's very alkalising and is good for flushing the liver.

1 teaspoon unpasteurised raw apple cider vinegar
1 teaspoon raw honey

Simply boil your kettle, fill your tea cup and let it sit for a minute or two to cool, then stir in the vinegar and honey. By allowing the water to cool a little you will not be destroying the health properties of the vinegar and honey. Stir and drink.

MINT & ORANGE BLOSSOM TEA

Both mint and orange are uplifting so this will elevate your mood and bring general cheer. It's also cleansing and delicious.

6 fresh or dried mint leaves
6 fresh or dried orange blossoms
raw honey to taste (optional)

Place the herb leaves and flowers into a large teapot and pour over boiling water.

Allow to steep for 6-7 minutes. You can add honey if you like, to taste. I prefer it without, but that's just me...

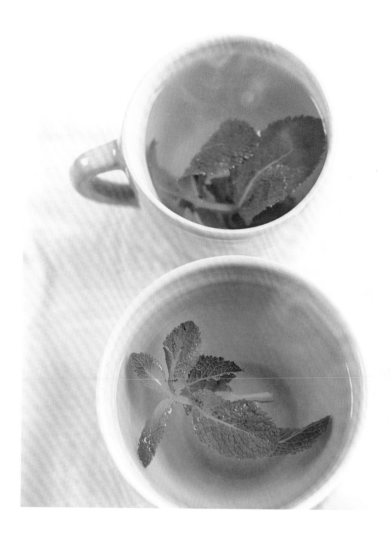

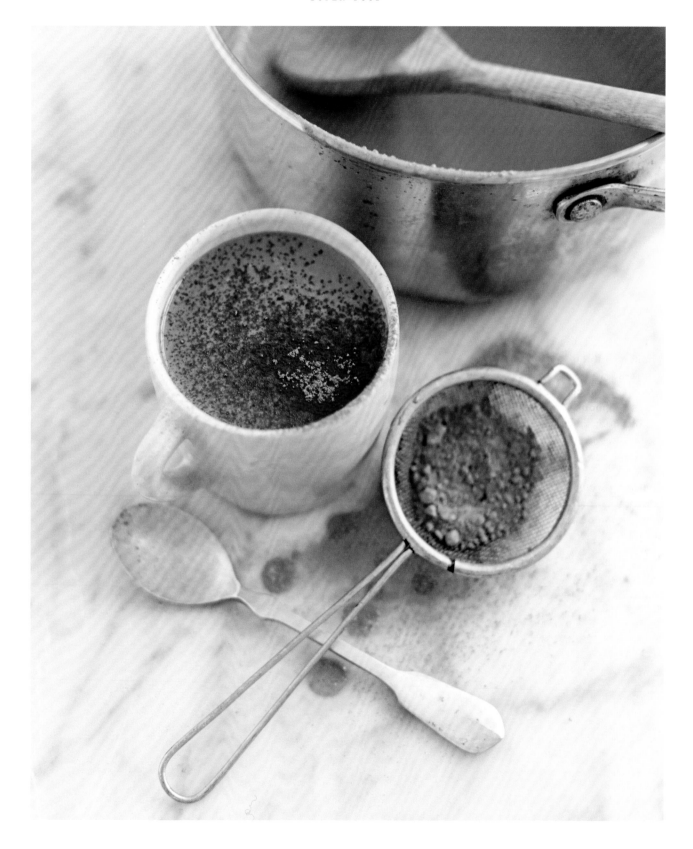

Very delicious

HOT CHOCOLATE

This delicious hot chocolate has all the allure and taste of a hot chocolate but without any of the nasties of the more conventional sugar laden type. It has cacao, which is FULL of mood enhancing properties and wonderful antioxidants. It's full of healthy fats, which feed the brain and give energy with out being stored. It has natural sweetening and above all it is still comforting and delicious and such a treat for a rainy cold day when a blanket and a cosy spot with a mug of this is the only thing that will give warmth and deliciousness.

Small handful of cashew nuts, soaked in filtered water for a few hours or overnight
400ml full-fat coconut milk
1½ tablespoons raw cacao powder
1 tablespoon raw honey or raw date syrup (or to taste – you can add more after it is heated if you want it sweeter)

Optional flavourings:
Pinch of cinnamon
¼ teaspoon orange peel zest
or
¼ teaspoon vanilla powder
or
Pinch of chilli and a pinch of cinnamon

Drain and rinse the soaked cashew nuts.

Throw everything into a blender, including the extra spices if you fancy. Blitz until you have a smooth liquid.

Pour it into a saucepan and place over a gentle heat until it reaches a good temperature. Check the sweetness and add more honey or date syrup if you wish.

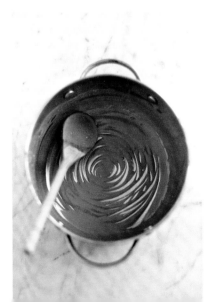

CUCUMBER, MINT, LIME & KIWI WATER

This is a cleansing, refreshing way to get your fluids in the hot summer months. You can prepare this the night before so it's ready the next morning. To make it extra cold, just add a handful of ice.

½ **cucumber, washed and sliced**
6 **sprigs mint, washed**
3 **limes, unwaxed, washed and sliced**
2 **kiwi fruit, peeled and sliced**
2l **pure spring or mineral water
or freshly filtered water**

Put all the ingredients into a large jug and allow to sit in a cool place or the fridge for at least 30 minutes.

RED SUMMER BERRIES

with Lemon & Rose

This is such a beautiful way to drink water, infused with the scent of rose and strawberries and the taste of lemon. It has extra cleansing properties from the lemon and berries. It's best drunk within one day, but, if I'm really thirsty or sharing this with others, I drink all the water and then keep topping it up throughout the day. You can add ice to keep it cool.

300g **mixed red berries
(strawberries and raspberries)**
2 **lemons, unwaxed, washed and sliced**
2 **big garden roses, washed and petals removed
(must be unsprayed)**
2l **pure spring or mineral water
or freshly filtered water**

Put all the ingredients into a large jug and allow to sit in a cool place or the fridge for at least 30 minutes, or make this the night before so it's ready to go the next morning.

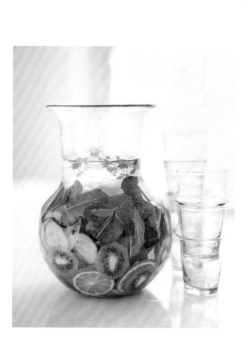

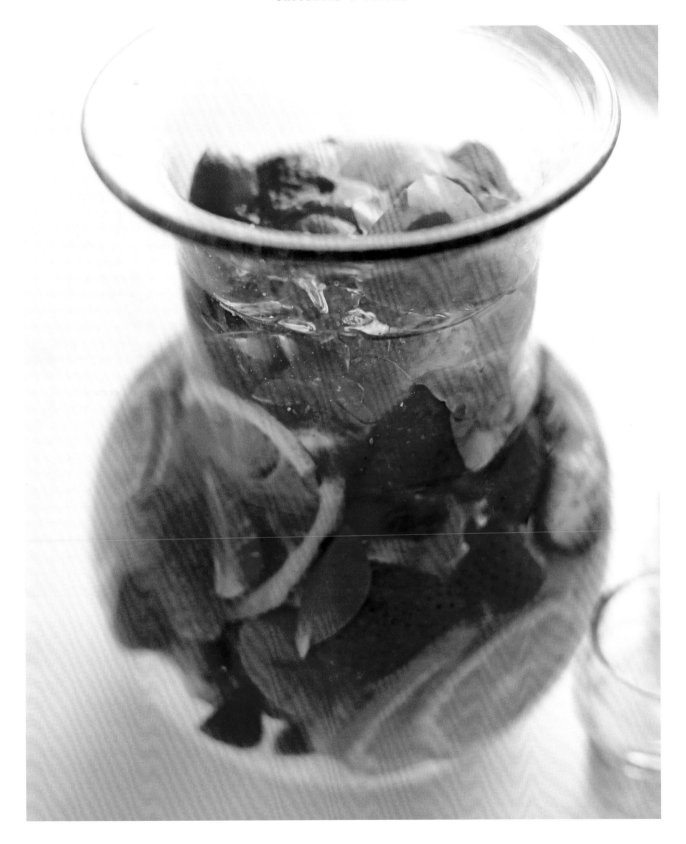

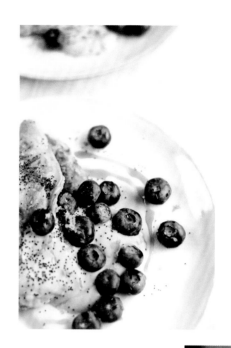

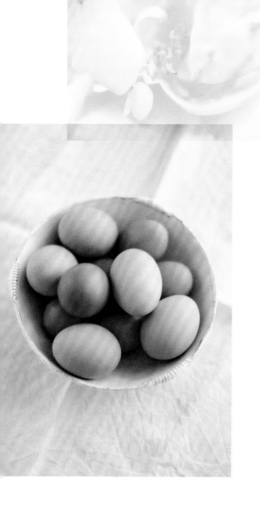

TO START THE DAY

breakfast

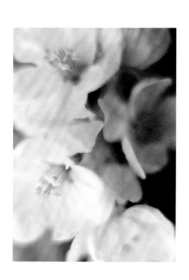

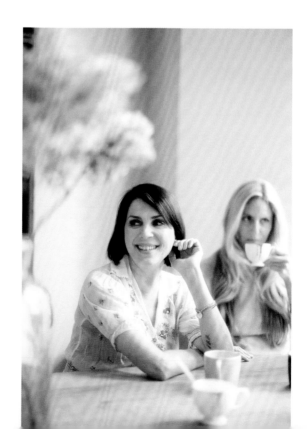

Breakfasts are often the highlight of my day. I am a HUGE breakfast fan, and love everything from making my own granolas to pancakes and healthy fry-ups (if you can believe it's possible, which it is!!!). My son LOVES his breakfasts too. During the week, I try to be organised and have some kind of seasonal fruit compôte in the fridge that I can add to porridge or to yoghurt and granola. Whether it's a quick weekday start or a leisurely weekend affair, there is every reason to prepare something beautiful, seasonal, delicious and nutrient-dense. In this chapter, I hope you will find lots of inspiration and new ideas to try out.

LEMON & POPPYSEED
SWEET OMELETTE

Here's a refreshing way to start any day! The tart lemon lifts and adds a brightness, the poppyseeds provide a tasty little crunch and what could be better than maple syrup and berries? The omelette is grain-free and full of essential good fats to feed your brain for a busy day ahead. It can easily be dairy-free if you use coconut yoghurt, which is so good for you and utterly delicious.

Serves 1
2 free-range eggs
Pinch of good salt
1 generous teaspoon maple syrup,
  plus extra for drizzling
Zest of ¼ of an unwaxed lemon,
  plus extra to serve
1 teaspoon poppyseeds
1 heaped teaspoon coconut oil

To serve
1 generous dollop of your favourite yoghurt
1 small handful of fresh blueberries

Place a small frying pan over a medium-high heat. Break the eggs into a small bowl and whisk thoroughly until they are very light and fluffy: the fluffier the eggs, the fluffier your omelette. Mix in the salt, syrup, lemon zest and half the poppyseeds.

Add the coconut oil to the hot pan, let it cover the base and use a flat wooden spatula to spread it around, then pour in your mix. Carefully pull in the sides with the spatula while tilting the pan and then let the egg run back out to fill the gap. Continue in this fashion until there is no runny mix left. Now carefully flip the omelette over – the second side will only need 30 seconds or so.

Gently slide the omelette out of the pan onto a waiting plate, spoon over your fave yoghurt and top with blueberries, a final drizzle of maple syrup and sprinkle on the remaining poppyseeds and some lemon zest. Enjoy while hot.

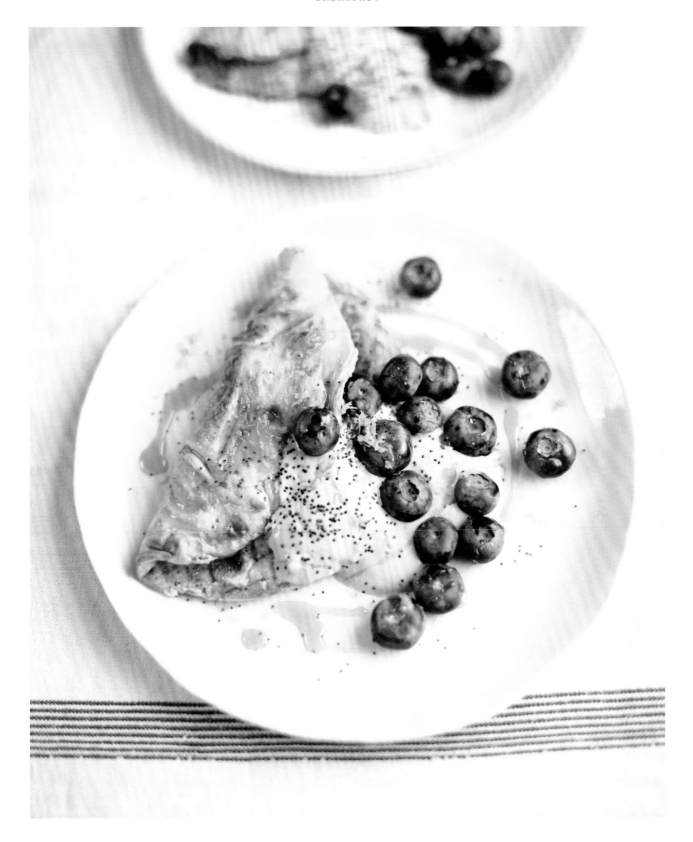

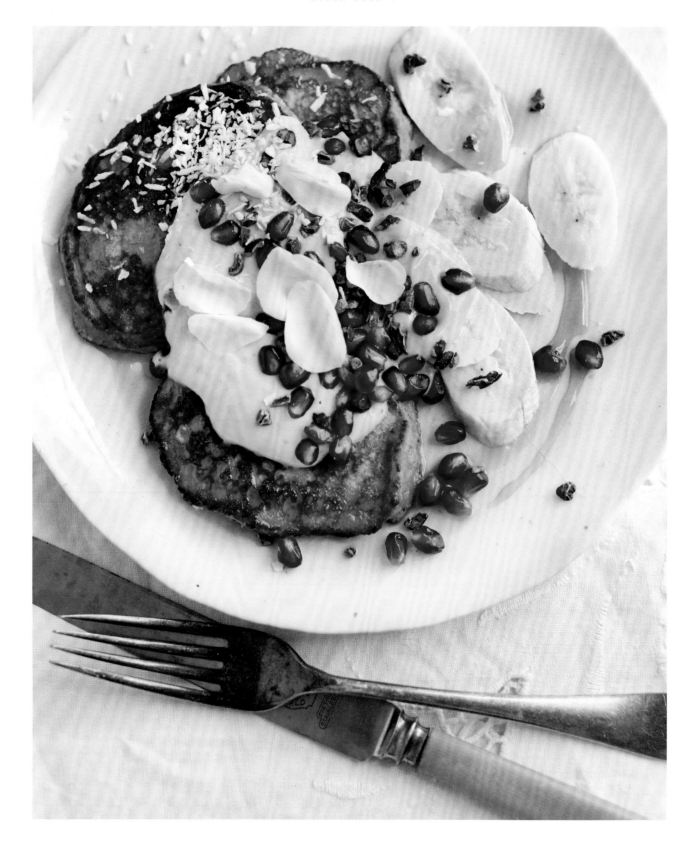

COCONUT &
BANANA PANCAKES

I love pancakes (who doesn't?)! These little ones are great topped with fresh fruit and yoghurt for breakfast or brunch, or served as an afternoon tea much like drop scones with cream and jam. Sounds naughty but it needn't be, if you have organic cream or whipped coconut cream sweetened with honey and a fresh sugar-free berry fridge jam then everything is good for you and totally nourishing.

Serves 2–3
2 ripe medium bananas, roughly chopped
4 whole eggs
2 tablespoons honey
70g desiccated coconut
100g almond meal
½ teaspoon gluten-free baking powder
Ghee or coconut oil for cooking

To serve
A few spoonfuls of your favourite yoghurt
Handful of your favourite seasonal fruit
Toasted coconut or cacao nibs

Put the bananas, eggs and honey in a food processor and purée until light and fluffy (or use a bowl and a stick blender). Add the coconut, almond meal and baking powder and beat to combine.

Heat up a tiny amount of coconut oil or ghee in your frying pan over a low to medium heat. Cook in batches, allowing a biggish spoonful of mix per pancake – too big and they are really hard to flip, so keep them drop-scone size. Cook thoroughly – they should take about 1½ minutes on each side; you will know when to flip them once little bubbles start to appear on the surface. Keep warm and continue to cook the rest of the batter, adding a little more oil to the pan between batches.

Serve while hot and delicious with some of your favourite toppings.

POACHED EGGS

*with Cauliflower Toasts,
Kale & Dukkah*

*This delicious ensemble is a serious treat, one of my all-time favourites. Cauliflower toasts
give the poached eggs something to sit on and add texture without the need for bread.*

Serves 2

1 whole cauliflower, outer leaves removed, washed
3 tablespoons cold-pressed olive oil
2 tablespoons Dukkah (see page 115) or lightly
   crushed cumin seeds, plus extra to serve
2 tablespoons cold-pressed olive oil
1 tablespoon butter
2 garlic cloves, thinly sliced
½ medium red chilli (optional), finely sliced
6–8 kale or cavolo nero leaves, on the large side,
   washed and centre stalks stripped out
4 free-range eggs
Salt

To serve
Cold-pressed extra virgin olive oil
Juice of ½ lemon
A few twists of pepper

Preheat the oven to 200°C/gas mark 6 and line a baking tray with baking paper. Cut the cauliflower across into 4 slices of 'toast' about 1.5–2cm thick. Drizzle with some of the oil, sprinkle with dukkah, place the toasts on your tray and pop into the oven for about 30 minutes until they start to turn lovely and golden.

After 20 minutes, melt the oil and butter in a medium, lidded casserole over a medium heat. Add the garlic and chilli (if using), stir for 30 seconds, add the kale then a few tablespoons of water and a pinch of salt. Cover tightly with the lid and braise for 10 minutes, stirring occasionally. You may need to turn the heat down or add a little extra water if it is cooking too furiously.

Place a wide casserole style dish over a high heat and fill it with boiling water from the kettle. Bring it to a light simmer and add a pinch of salt. Carefully crack one egg into a cup then gently pour it into the simmering water. Repeat with the remaining eggs and cook to your liking. Depending on their size, a soft poached egg takes about 2 minutes and a soft to firm one needs about 4 minutes.

When everything is ready, place the cauliflower toasts onto warm plates, top with the eggs and place the kale alongside. Sprinkle over a little extra dukkah, give a drizzle of cold-pressed extra virgin olive oil, a squeeze of lemon over the kale and a few twists of pepper.

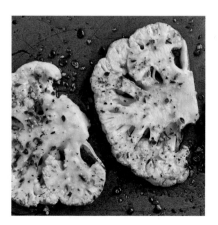

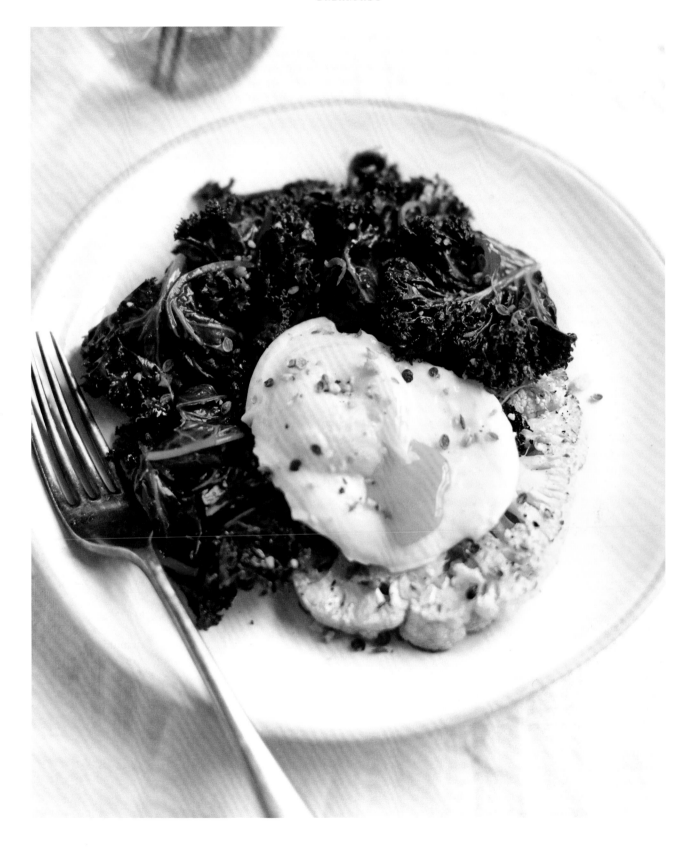

ONE PLAIN OMELETTE

You can add any number of things, to make it into something filling and satisfying. One of my favourite ways to serve an omelette is with plenty of sorrel. Sorrel is full of calcium and magnesium - two things we could all do with more of. I love the sourness of sorrel. Omelettes go well with roast sweet potato or squash and a green salad, or anything green for that matter. Steamed greens work well with plenty of good grass-fed butter and some quality sea salt.

Serves 1
Small knob of butter or odourless coconut oil
2 eggs, lightly beaten
Sea salt flakes and freshly cracked black pepper

A few good things to have with an omelette:
• **A few slices of fresh avocado**
• **A sprinkle of your favourite herb**
• **Cheese, grated onto the omelette just before
  you fold it in half**
• **Radish Salad with Lemon and Parsley (see page 53)**
• **A few cherry tomatoes pan-fried
  with butter and thyme**
• **Any kind of steamed green: kale, broccoli, beans etc**
• **A few green leaves – kale or cos, lightly dressed
  with lemon juice and olive oil**
• **Baby spinach, wilted in a hot pan with a tiny
  bit of butter or oil**
• **A sprinkle of dukkah (see page 115)**

Add your knob of butter to the pan and as soon as it sizzles pour in the egg. Carefully tilt the pan and use a flat wooden spatula to pull in the sides of the omelette and then let it go – the egg will run back out to the sides filling the gap. Do this a few times around the pan, then let it cook for a few moments. When nearly all the egg is set, gently flip-fold over one side envelope fashion, scrape it onto a waiting plate and eat immediately.

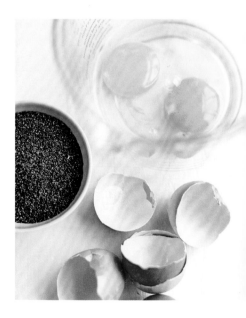

PORRIDGE

with Fresh Summer Berries, Lemon Zest,
Maple Syrup & Toasted Coconut

Although porridge is generally thought of as a warming breakfast for winter, I sometimes enjoy it as a summer dish too, served with fresh fruit, which makes it lighter, and summer berries add a zingy, fresh taste. This is totally scrumptious and very nourishing.

Serves 2
100g whole rolled oats
480ml unsweetened almond milk
  or spring water
¼ teaspoon finely grated lemon zest
Pinch of salt

To serve
200g shredded coconut
Yoghurt of choice
2 big handfuls of summer berries
  of your choice (I like to use
  blueberries and raspberries)
Maple syrup to taste

First toast your coconut. Place a largish frying pan over a medium heat and let it warm up for a few minutes until you can feel the heat coming off the pan. Tip in the coconut and stir constantly with a wooden spoon. Slowly, it will start to turn a lovely golden brown but, if it doesn't start to colour, you need to turn up the heat. Once it's golden and smells delicious, tip it into a waiting bowl to cool.

To make your porridge, put the oats, milk or water, lemon zest and salt into a saucepan and place over a medium-high heat and bring to the boil. Once it bubbles, stir constantly with a wooden spoon for 5–6 minutes. Remove the pan from the heat and divide between 2 bowls.

Serve with a generous dollop of your favourite yoghurt then scatter over the fresh berries, drizzle over the maple syrup and top with the toasted coconut. Enjoy.

BUCKWHEAT PORRIDGE

with Cinnamon & Sultanas

This is just the thing to keep you nourished and balanced and it's a bowl of such delicious flavours you'll be in breakfast heaven – I sometimes even have this for dessert. Blackberries and pears are the perfect fruit combination for autumn and winter as they're full of antioxidants, gentle on the digestive system and yet full of fibre, vitamins C and E and other essential nutrients. Cinnamon is a warming spice, great for curbing sugar cravings and the thyme adds a delicious sweet note. Despite its name, buckwheat is technically not a grain but a seed. It is gluten-free with a lovely nutty flavour and it has a natural affinity to pears.

Serves 2

200g buckwheat groats
¼ teaspoon cinnamon
Small handful of sultanas
Small handful of blackberries
230ml spring water
480ml unsweetened almond milk,
  or your favourite raw milk
Pinch of good salt

To serve
2 big dollops of yoghurt of your choice
1 ripe pear, peeled, cored and sliced
  lengthways into quarters
Maple syrup to taste
Small handful of roasted and roughly
  chopped almonds
A few sprigs of thyme (optional but delicious)

Put the buckwheat groats, cinnamon, sultanas and blackberries in a saucepan with the water, bring to the boil and then reduce the heat to a very gentle simmer. As the groats start to absorb the water stir in half the almond milk. Cover with a lid and allow the groats to absorb more of the liquid. You will need to stir the pan regularly with a wooden spoon and, when the groats have absorbed almost all the milk, add the rest of the almond milk and a pinch of salt, stir thoroughly, replace the lid and allow them to absorb the rest of the liquid. The whole process should take 20–30 minutes – you may need to add a little more liquid if the groats start to dry out before they have finished cooking, so keep an eye on the pan.

When it is ready, divide the porridge between two bowls, top with yoghurt and the pear quarters then drizzle with maple syrup and sprinkle with the chopped almonds and some thyme if you wish.

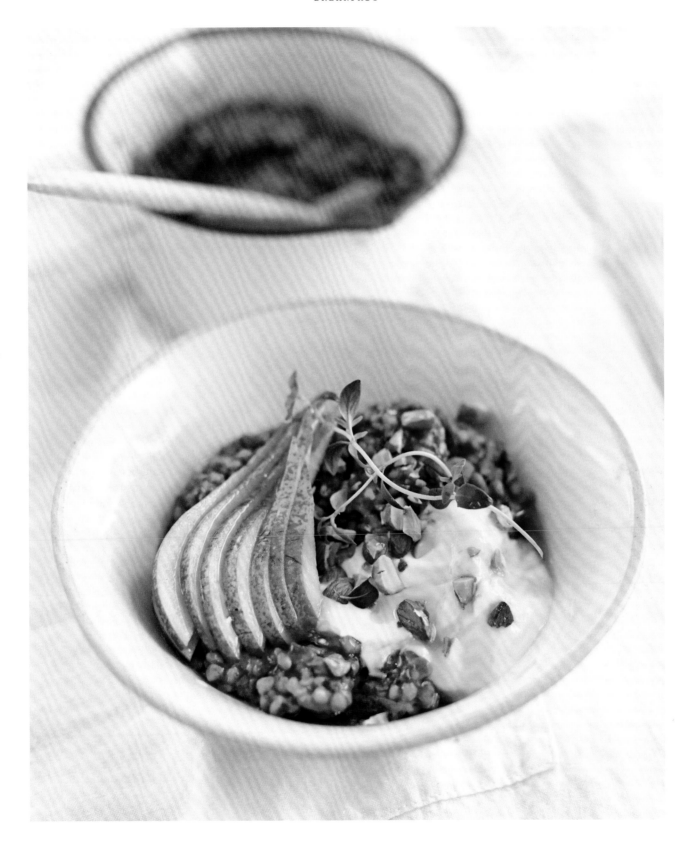

GRANOLA

Grain-free with Rosewater,
Apricot & Pistachio

This is a heavenly, fruity, floral combination. It's quite a decadent granola and not cheap to make; however, it lasts a long time and is not the kind of granola you would have a huge bowl of. I tend to serve it with fresh fruit and yoghurt, or a smoothie bowl, and then sprinkle the granola on top. It looks so pretty and adds crunch and flavour to what you serve it with. It's full of slow release energy and is super easy to make.

Makes 1 large jar
50g raw coconut oil
80ml honey
85ml maple syrup
200g coconut chips
115g pistachio nuts, roughly chopped
150g almonds, very roughly chopped
80g sunflower seeds
80g pumpkin seeds
1 teaspoon rosewater
200g dried apricots, roughly chopped
2 tablespoons hemp seeds
2–3 tablespoons dried rose petals (optional)

Preheat the oven to 170°C/gas mark 3 and line 2 deep-sided baking trays with baking parchment. Melt the coconut oil, honey and maple syrup in a small saucepan until it starts to bubble and simmer, then turn off the heat.

Combine the coconut chips, pistachio nuts, almonds, sunflower and pumpkin seeds in a largish bowl. Pour in the honey mixture, and stir with a wooden spoon until thoroughly combined. There should be enough of the honey mixture to lightly coat all the dry mix, but if you feel there is not enough just add more honey mix using equal amounts of melted honey and coconut oil.

Spread the mixture onto the lined baking trays, making a layer that isn't too deep, otherwise it won't all crisp up. Bake for 15–20 minutes, stirring every 3–4 minutes so that all the mix turns a lovely golden colour and doesn't burn, which it can do easily due to the coconut. Remove from the oven, allow to cool a little then sprinkle over the rosewater, if using, and scatter in the dried apricots and hemp seeds. Lastly stir through the petals.

Allow to cool completely before transferring into an airtight jar. Use within two weeks.

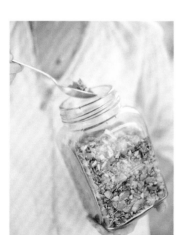

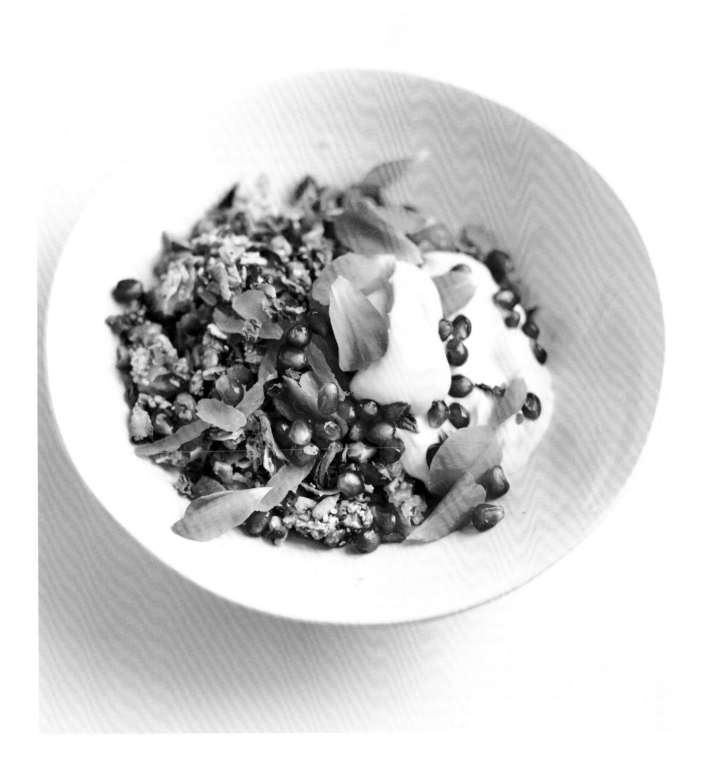

MY NOURISHING OVERNIGHT BERRY & CHIA PARFAIT

This makes a great breakfast, sooo delicious and it will give you a bumper start to the day. I don't always like to eat first thing so sometimes, with an early start to work, this is an ideal way to have a healthy breakfast on the go. Sometimes I make this the night before and put it in the fridge in a small jar which has a tight-fitting lid, allowing enough room at the top to add yoghurt and fruit once the parfait has set. That makes it really easy to have breakfast to go.

If you want to really go to town with this, layer it in a beautiful glass, starting with a layer of the parfait, followed by a layer of yoghurt then a layer of fruit then a sprinkling of Granola (see page 40). The kids like to get involved in this, too.

Serves 2
For the parfait
350ml of your favourite milk
100g dark berries (use a mix of blackcurrants, raspberries, strawberries and blueberries)
6 tablespoons chia seeds
1 tablespoon raw coconut oil
Drizzle of maple syrup or raw honey
1 tablespoon raw coconut oil (optional)

To serve (any or all of the following)
Small handful of fresh berries
Your favourite yoghurt
Seeds from ½ pomegranate
2 tablespoons shelled hemp seeds
Cacao nibs
Chopped nuts

Put all the ingredients for the parfait into a blender and blitz until thoroughly combined. Spoon one third of the mixture into the bottom of a glass and another third into the bottom of a second glass and the remaining third into a spare small container. Put all three in the fridge to set overnight.

When you are ready to eat this glass of delicious goodness, take both glasses from the fridge, sprinkle over some berries, then layer some yoghurt, then half the remaining third chia parfait into each glass. Top with more fresh fruit and any of the suggested toppings.

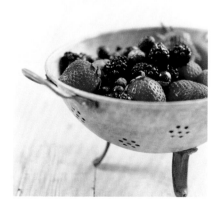

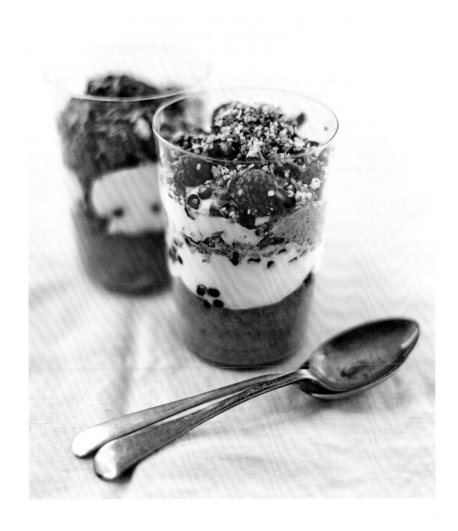

AVOCADO, BASIL
& CHILLI ON TOAST

This has to be one of my easiest and yet most delicious recipes. It's certainly one that I make most frequently – for breakfast, brunch (with a poached egg), lunch (with 2 eggs) and sometimes for dinner when I can't be bothered to cook… It's AMAZING sprinkled with a little dukkah; it's so good for you – full of healthy fats and essential micro nutrients that support your immune system and general health.

Serves 2
1 avocado
¼ teaspoon chilli flakes
6 basil leaves, washed and torn
3 tablespoons really good extra virgin olive oil
Squeeze of lemon juice
Sea salt and freshly ground black pepper

A couple of slices of your fave toast – perhaps
    sourdough rye
    or Cauliflower Toasts (see page 34)
1 garlic clove, halved
2 tablespoons good olive oil

To serve
Dukkah (see page 115), optional

Slice the avocado in half and remove the pit. Use a small sharp knife to slice the inside of the avocado into large squares without cutting into the skin. Now take a spoon and scoop out the squares and put them in a bowl, along with the chilli flakes, torn basil leaves and oil. Squeeze over the lemon, add some salt and pepper to taste and give it a good but gentle stir – you don't want mush.

Toast the bread, and rub it all over with half a garlic clove – I like it quite garlicky but if you prefer it less so just give a very light rub with the garlic. Drizzle with some good oil and sprinkle over a little sea salt and a few twists of pepper. Top with the avocado and serve.

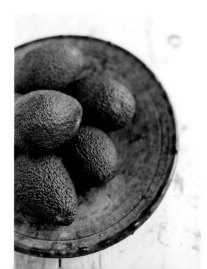

MY SPICE-SCENTED
HOMEMADE BEANS ON TOAST

I love beans on toast, and this is a version that I've been making for years. Kids love it too. Either serve them simply as beans on a nice piece of toasted sourdough rye or on the cauliflower toasts (see page 34) if you want to go grain-free, or with some lightly steamed kale, a delicious soft-poached egg, roasted veg – you name it…

Serves 4–6

3 tablespoons cold-pressed olive oil
2 medium onions, roughly chopped
2 garlic cloves, grated or finely chopped
½ teaspoon ground cumin
½ teaspoon whole cumin seeds
1 x 400g tin chopped tomatoes
1 tablespoon tomato purée
70g maple syrup
80ml apple cider vinegar
250ml water
2 x 400g tins white beans
  (cannellini or butter beans), rinsed and drained
Salt and pepper to taste

To serve
A few sprigs of fresh coriander
½ medium red chilli, deseeded and finely sliced
A few slices of your favourite cheese

Heat the oil in a large, heavy-based casserole or saucepan, add the onion, garlic and cumin, and stir for 3–5 minutes or until the onion is translucent and softened.

Add the tinned tomatoes, the purée, syrup, vinegar and water. Bring to the boil, add the beans, reduce the heat to very low and leave to simmer gently, uncovered, for about 1.5 hours: you will need to stir the beans regularly and add more water if they are drying out. After this time the beans should be lovely and soft and the sauce wonderfully thick. Season to taste.

Sometimes, if I am feeling really decadent, I add a few shavings of my favourite cheese or sprinkle some fresh coriander and fresh chilli on top. Whatever you decide, enjoy this while it's lovely and hot.

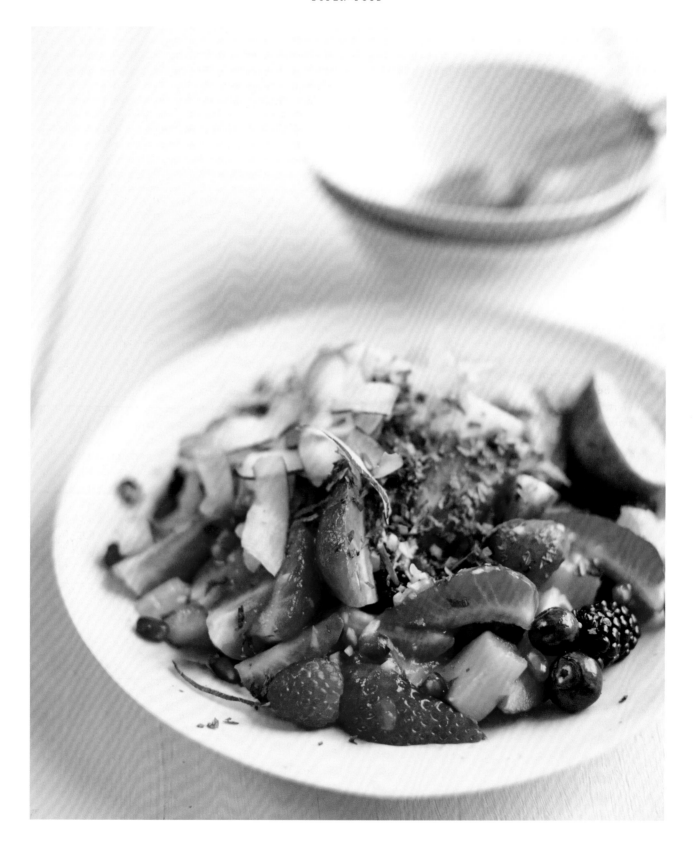

SOM TUM POLLAMAI

Seasonal Fruit Salad with
Thai Herbs & Fresh Lime Juice

*This is a really tasty way of making fruit salad known as Som Tum Pollamai in
Thailand. The Thai herbs make it very fresh, zesty and quite different. You can use
any fruits but the ones I have chosen here are some of the most nutrient-rich of
their type. Granny smith apples have been found to contain up to 17 times more
phyto nutrients than other apple varieties. Dark-coloured berries have increased
amounts of anthocyanins, which are powerful antioxidants.*

Serves 4
1 granny smith apple, washed, unpeeled, halved,
  cored and sliced into half moons
300g dark berries (choose from blueberries,
  blackberries, strawberries, raspberries,
  boysenberries or red grapes)
2 white-fleshed peaches or nectarines,
  washed and sliced
1 mango, peeled and sliced or diced
Seeds from ½ pomegranate

3 tablespoons raw date syrup or raw honey
2 tablespoons freshly squeezed lime juice
¼ teaspoon sea salt
1 tablespoon very finely chopped lemongrass
8–10 fresh mint leaves, finely chopped
Zest of 1 lime

To serve
Handful of coconut flakes,
  lightly toasted in the oven
Fresh yoghurt
  (coconut yoghurt would be very good
  if you can find it)

Put all the prepared fruit in a bowl. Combine the
date syrup, lime juice and salt in another bowl. Stir,
pour over the fruit, and toss well. Allow the fruit to sit
for 5 minutes. Just before serving, add the chopped
lemongrass, mint and lime zest.

Scoop into bowls, top with coconut flakes and yoghurt.
Eat when fresh.

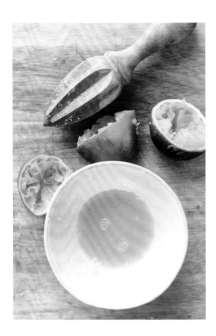

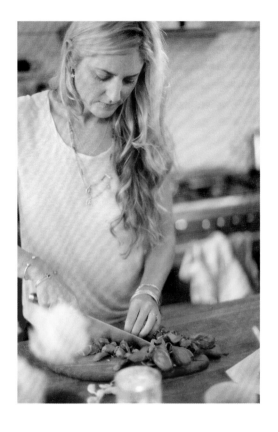

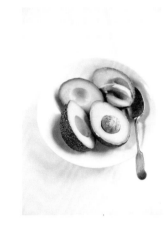

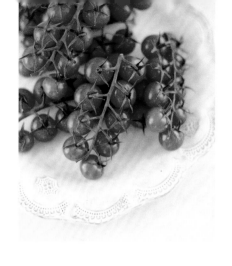

SOUPS
&
SALADS

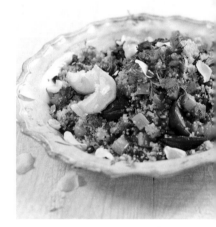

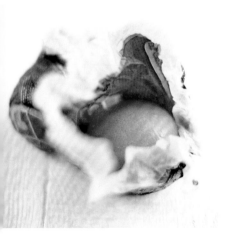

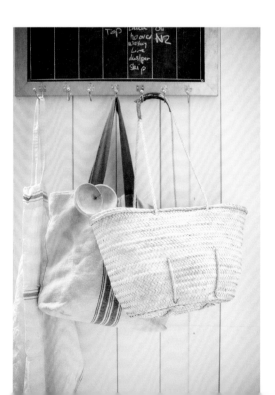

Here is a selection of dishes to get you through various seasons and moods. I have tried to keep the salads more of a side salad selection to go with the main dishes but you could always beef them up by adding a bit of this and a bit of that as I often do. I am always improvising and making things up as I go along, sometimes it's the best way. However if it's a little inspiration you need or some seasonal guidance then peek through this chapter for some delicicous ideas. I tend to make my salad and soup recipes with flexibility in mind so that you could rustle them up for a lunch or a dinner, by adding other things. Sometimes there is nothing nicer than a simple radish salad with a beautiful piece of fresh soft cheese and a squeeze of lemon and some fresh herbs, lending their greenness and bite. With simple recipes I wanted to show you how easy it is to rustle up something healthy and really lovely and yummy.

CHICKEN SOUP

For the Soul (two ways)

*This soup is pretty much foolproof and in terms of health benefits it's liquid gold.
Whenever my son or I feel poorly I make a big batch and drink a cup of this broth
morning, noon and night. They don't call it Jewish penicillin for nothing! It really is the
most restorative, healing, soothing and nourishing thing you can drink.
I have shown the two ways I make it most; both are tasty.*

Makes 1 large pot serving 4–6
1 whole free-range organic chicken, washed
1 teaspoon black peppercorns
3 bay leaves
3 celery sticks, washed and cut into chunks
2 onions, peeled and quartered
2 garlic cloves, peeled
4 carrots, peeled and cut into chunks
3 tablespoons unfiltered apple cider vinegar
Handful of parsley
A few sprigs of thyme
Hearty pinch or two of sea salt

To serve
Either
**Bunch of purple or green curly kale, leaves
   stripped from stalks and chopped**
**Bunch of carrots, peeled, sliced thinly on
   the diagonal**
700–750g (roughly) cooked quinoa
juice of 1 lemon
3 tablespoons raw coconut oil
A few sprigs of thyme
Or
Knob of ginger, peeled and finely grated
Small bunch of mint
Small bunch of coriander
1 medium chilli, deseeded and finely sliced
juice of 1 lemon
3 tablespoons raw coconut oil

To make the bone broth, put everything for the soup into a really big stockpot and just cover it all with filtered water if possible, otherwise use tap water – the better the water the bigger the benefits.

Bring to the boil over a high heat, reduce the heat to a very light simmer, only just bubbling, then place the lid on and simmer for 3 hours. Let the stock cool a bit and then strain. Discard all but the chicken.

Remove all the meat from the bones in lovely big flakes, don't shred it. Transfer the cooled stock back into the pot along with the chicken meat.

At this point you will have chosen which flavours you want to add from the serving options. If using kale and carrots, add them to the pot, simmer for 10 minutes or until the carrots are tender, and taste for seasoning. Add the cooked quinoa to the pot, and let it sit for a minute. Ladle the soup into bowls, squeeze a little lemon juice over each one together with about ½ tablespoon of coconut oil and top with a sprig of thyme. Or, if using ginger, mint, coriander and chilli, simply add the grated ginger to the soup in the pot, reheat, taste for seasoning then ladle into bowls. Add a few leaves of each herb into the bowls and top with a few slices of chilli, a squeeze of lemon juice and ½ tablespoon of coconut oil. Serve hot.

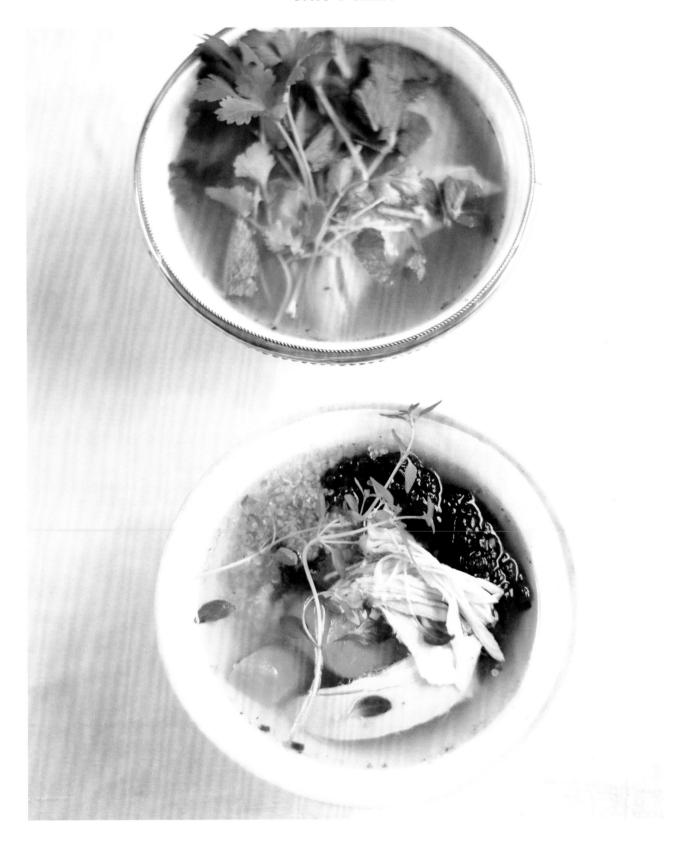

RUBY CHARD
SOUP

This is a simple soup; it's a light, summery one and a great way of using greens. You can use any kind of chard or even kale if you can't get your hands on the ruby chard. The light vegetable or chicken broth is very restorative, whilst also being full of flavour.

Makes 1 large pot
3 tablespoons cold-pressed sunflower oil or raw odourless coconut oil
1 large yellow onion, peeled and finely diced
8 stems (about) ruby chard, washed, stalks removed and sliced and leaves cut into 2.5cm strips
2 x 400g tins cannellini beans, rinsed and drained
2.5l vegetable or chicken stock
5-6 tablespoons chilli oil
salt and pepper to taste

Start by placing a large pot over a high heat, drizzle in your oil and then tip in the diced onion. Allow it to sizzle a bit then turn the heat down to low and sauté for about 5-6 minutes until the onion is translucent; you don't want it to colour. Add the ruby chard, leaves and stalks. Add the beans and then gently pour over the stock.

Simmer for about 20 minutes, remove from the heat and check seasoning.

Serve in warmed bowls, drizzled with the chilli oil.

BORLOTTI BEANS
with Artichoke Hearts

This little side is great with chicken or fish or roast veg. It goes spectacularly well with garlic aïoli and a piece of grilled white fish with herbs – a most heavenly combination.

Serves 4–6 as a side
10 roasted artichoke hearts in oil, with some of the oil
2 x 400g tins borlotti beans, rinsed and drained
Squeeze of lemon juice
Sea salt and freshly ground black pepper

Place a frying pan over quite a high heat and, while it is warming, slice the artichoke hearts into quarters and throw them into the pan along with a couple of tablespoons of the oil from the jar.

Add the beans and stir them carefully – you want the beans to stay as whole as possible. Cook them only as long as it takes for them to be hot through – this will take 2–3 minutes.

Spoon them into a lovely serving bowl and squeeze over a little lemon and sprinkle with a little sea salt and freshly ground black pepper.

RADISH SALAD

with Lemon & Parsley

For such a small vegetable, radishes really pack a serious punch in the health department. For a start, they cleanse the body and help it to eliminate toxins and free radicals, they soothe the digestive system, prevent viral infections and keep you hydrated.

Serves 4 as a side
600g round radishes, washed (the colourful ones are pretty if you can find them)
½ lemon
Olive oil
Sea salt and freshly ground black pepper
Small handful of parsley, washed and finely sliced

Simply slice all the radishes into thin little rounds, place them into a lovely bowl. Squeeze over some lemon juice, drizzle a little oil, scatter some salt and pepper. Lastly scatter over the parsley, give everything a good toss and serve.

PUY LENTILS

with Wilted Spinach

A delicious grain-free side – earthy, protein-rich lentils are sublime cooked with silky, buttery wilted spinach. Great with Roast Pumpkin, Golden Beets and Squash Salad (see page 59) and Hummus, or maybe a piece of fish or chicken and some homemade mayo (see page 111).

Serves 4
200g puy lentils
700ml chicken or veg stock or water
A few glugs of olive oil
Knob of butter
100g baby spinach
Sea salt and freshly ground black pepper

Rinse the lentils under running water and then put them into a large pot and cover with stock or water. Bring to the boil and simmer for 20–25 minutes – you want them with a bit of a bite, not mushy. Drain.

Put a large frying pan over a medium-high heat and add the drained lentils, oil and butter. Throw in your spinach and cook until just wilting – it will only take a minute. Season to taste and serve.

FENNEL SALAD

with Blood Oranges, Buffalo Mozzarella & Dill

This has to be one for special occasions, as blood oranges are only available for a short time. They are a joy to behold, and make a delicious pairing with the mozzarella, mint and fennel. This salad is cleansing and has a bright clean taste – I love it with roast chicken and a big green salad. It's delicious as a topping for a slice of toasted sourdough rye bread that has had a light rub with a garlic clove and a drizzle of oil ... so very good! Great for lunch or a merry get together as part of a dinner.

Serves 6

2 fennel bulbs, trimmed and washed

2 blood oranges, peeled to remove any of the outer white pith and membrane (use ordinary oranges when blood oranges are out of season)

2 balls of buffalo mozzarella

4 sprigs of dill, washed and leaves picked

4 tablespoons really good cold-pressed olive oil

Juice of ½ lemon

Sea salt and freshly cracked pepper

Start by taking a very thin slice off the very bottom of the fennel. This removes any brown bits and gives a nice flat base so that you can set the fennel upright to slice it. Now slice the fennel as thinly as you can.

Arrange the fennel and orange slices on a lovely shallow platter. Tear up the mozzarella into medium pieces and arrange over the orange and fennel. Scatter over the dill, then drizzle with the olive oil and squeeze over the juice from the lemon. Add a pinch of sea salt and a few twists of pepper. Enjoy.

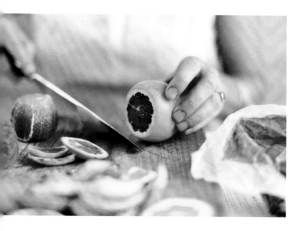

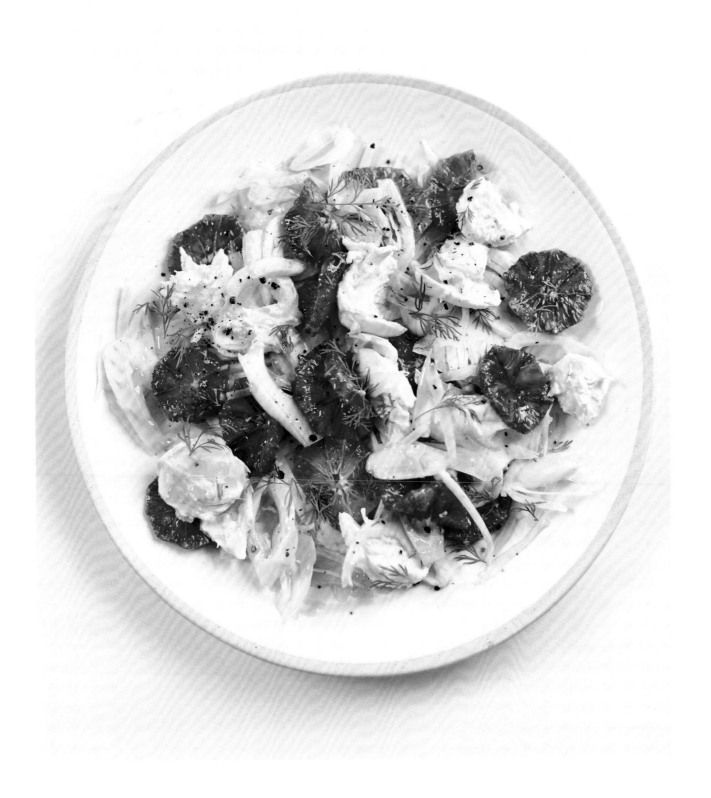

MY SMASHED CUCUMBER SALAD

This is a great way of using up an overflow of cucumbers, as can easily happen in the summertime, when the gardens are exploding. It is a delightful little salad, fresh and zingy, to accompany a barbecue if you're cooking meat or chicken. It's super cleansing and the enzymes, herbs and ginger help to digest richer food on the menu.

Serves 6
3 cucumbers, peeled
2 spring onions, sliced into thin rounds
½ green chilli, seeds removed, finely sliced
½ red chilli, seeds removed, finely sliced
5 teaspoons finely chopped mint leaves (or shiso leaves if you can find them)
4 teaspoons finely chopped coriander leaves
Sea salt and freshly ground black pepper

For the dressing
1 garlic clove, finely grated
5cm piece of ginger, peeled, finely grated
35ml apple cider vinegar
1½ teaspoons maple syrup
2 teaspoons toasted sesame oil
Pinch of sea salt

To make the dressing, combine the garlic, ginger, vinegar, syrup and oil. Give it a good whisk and then add a pinch of salt.

Cut the cucumbers into 6cm chunks then crush them using the flat blade of a large knife. Throw them into a bowl, add the spring onions, chillies, mint and coriander leaves, a pinch of salt and a few twists of pepper. Add the dressing, toss well, and serve.

PARSNIP *with* PARMESAN HASH

This is true comfort food, which is quick and really easy to make. It's also a different way of using parsnips; they're almost more delicious done this way than roasted. Great with an egg for breakfast or as a side for lunch or dinner.

Serves 4
3 tablespoons extra virgin olive oil
2 medium baking potatoes, scrubbed clean, halved lengthwise then thinly sliced into half moons
2 parsnips, peeled, halved lengthwise then thinly sliced into half moons
1 small onion, finely minced
50g shaved Parmesan Parmigiano-Reggiano
Sea salt and freshly ground black pepper

Preheat a large nonstick pan over a medium-high heat and add the oil. Add the potatoes and parsnips with a little seasoning and stir for 10–12 minutes or until the veg are cooked through and nicely coloured. Add the onion and continue cooking until everything is golden. Remove from the heat and stir through the Parmesan. Taste for seasoning and serve.

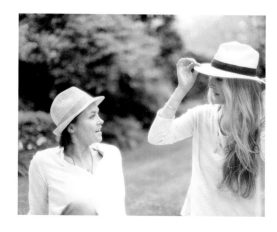

ROAST FENNEL

with Cherry Tomatoes

My rule is, if it's to be eaten raw, slice it as thinly as possible and, if you're cooking it, do it gently with lots of butter and good oils. Also, fennel LOVES lemon, so add lots of zest whether you're serving it raw or cooked. This is perfect as a bed for a little roasted red mullet or it would go beautifully with some quinoa (see page 62) and garlicky mayo (see page 111). Heaven.

Serves 6
3 fennel bulbs
20g butter (or if you don't want to use butter just use extra oil)
Zest and juice of ½ lemon
A few good glugs of olive oil
200g cherry tomatoes, preferably on the vine
Sea salt and freshly ground black pepper

Preheat the oven to 180°C/gas mark 4. Trim the bases off your fennel and tidy up the tops, removing any feathery leaves that don't look good to eat. Slice the fennel lengthways into wedges – depending on the size of the bulb I usually cut each half into 3 wedges. Lay the wedges in a baking dish, dot a few pieces of butter (if using) over the top, sprinkle over the zest and drizzle with oil.

Transfer to the oven and bake for 25 minutes. Place the cherry tomatoes on top of the cooking fennel and put the dish back in the oven for a further 15 minutes or until the tomatoes are starting to collapse and the skins are deliciously split with a bit of colour.

Squeeze over the lemon juice and sprinkle with a little salt and pepper.

MY FAVOURITE MASH

This is my favourite mash. I totally prefer it to mashed potato, which I find can be a bit boring. And I'm pretty sure once you've tried this colourful version you won't want conventional mash either! It's earthy, creamy, nourishing and delicious – and it goes with pretty much anything. Top with snipped chives.

Serves 4
125g parsnips, peeled and cut into chunks
250g sweet potato, peeled and cut into chunks
400g butternut squash, peeled and cut into chunks
100ml milk
Bay leaf
½ teaspoon finely grated or ground nutmeg
50g butter
Sea salt and freshly ground black pepper
3 tablespoons roughly chopped chives

Keep the parsnips separate from the sweet potato and squash. Put the parsnips in a small saucepan with the milk, bay leaf and nutmeg and cook until tender. Put the sweet potato and butternut squash in a second pan of salted water and cook until tender.

Drain all the veg, reserving the milk from the parsnips. Spread the veg onto a flat tray, again keeping the parsnips separate, and allow everything to dry off for a couple of minutes.

Tip the parsnips into a bowl and blitz with a stick blender. Add a knob of the butter and enough milk to give a smooth finish. Warm the remaining milk and butter in the saucepan you used to cook the veg, add the potato and squash and mash in the pan, off the heat, until smooth. Add the parsnip and stir well. Scoop into a serving bowl and sprinkle with chives.

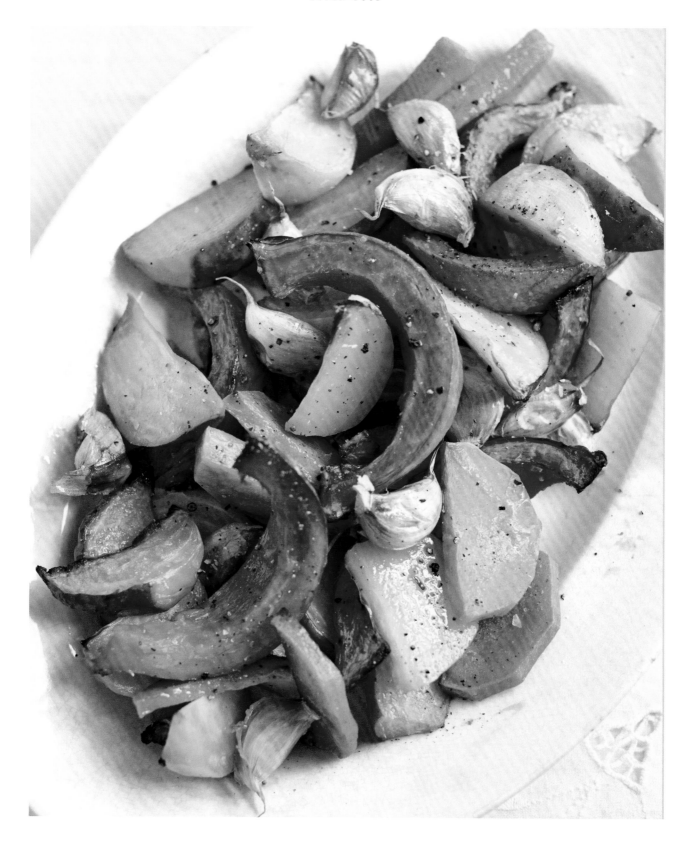

ROAST PUMPKIN, GOLDEN BEETS & SQUASH

with Rose Garlic

This warm salad is seriously nourishing, and the silky squash, earthy beets and the potent garlic combined make a flavoursome dish that you will love. It's super easy and looks colourful. It's great with some hummus and greens for lunch or as a side to something more substantial for dinner.

Serves 8

½ **butternut squash, washed, halved lengthways, seeds removed**

4 **golden beets, washed, peeled and cut into 6 wedges**

1 **medium orange pumpkin (acorn squash or Japanese red kuri), washed, halved, seeds removed**

1 **whole bulb rose garlic, cloves separated but unpeeled**

A few good glugs of olive oil

Sea salt and freshly ground pepper

Preheat the oven to 180°C/gas mark 4. Slice the butternut squash into 4 long slices and place on a big baking tray with the golden beet wedges. Cut the pumpkin halves into lovely crescent moon wedges – roughly 4 wedges per half pumpkin – and scatter those on the tray too with the garlic cloves.

Drizzle olive oil generously over everything, sprinkle with sea salt and pepper and roast in the oven for about 30–35 minutes. Keep an eye on them; you want the edges to start browning and the veg to be tender all the way through – check by inserting a small sharp knife into a thick piece.

Remove the veg from the oven and allow to cool a little. Transfer everything to a shallow platter and serve.

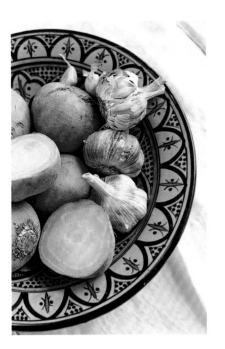

KALE

with Lemon & Caramelised Red Onions

You could also try this with cavalo nero, if you can find it. Apart from tasting amazing, both curly kale and cavolo nero are full of vitamins K and A as well as significant amounts of manganese, copper, fibre, calcium, iron and B vitamins and much else too. They're incredibly restorative and nourishing and a great source of fibre. Cooked with sweet onions and sharpened with a squeeze of lemon at the end to bring it all to life.

Serves 4

10–12 stems kale (or you can use cavalo nero)
Big knob of butter, or 1 tablespoon odourless raw coconut oil
Generous drizzle of olive oil
1 large red onion, halved, peeled and sliced into thin half moons
Juice of ½ lemon
Sea salt and freshly ground black pepper

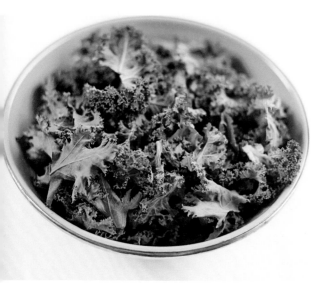

Put a large, lidded frying pan over a high heat. While it's warming, give the kale or cavolo a quick rinse and then strip the central stalks away from the leafy green bits. Discard the tough stalks (good for the bunnies).
Put the butter and olive oil into the hot pan and, when it sizzles, add your onion and turn down the heat to medium/low, stirring the onions all the time – you don't want them to catch. After 8 minutes they should be soft and sweet.

Throw in the kale or cavolo and about 20ml of water – just enough to steam the veg a little – and cover with the lid; the water will evaporate as the leaves cook, provided you don't add too much.

A couple of minutes later lift the lid and stir. You may need to turn up the heat again if it's not bubbling and steaming: keep an eye on it. It needs to cook for about 4–5 minutes. If the pan dries out too much and is catching add another small knob of butter.

When everything is lovely and cooked and smelling delicious take the pan off the heat, add a sprinkle of salt, a few twists of pepper then squeeze over your lemon. Serve.

STEAMED VEG

Japanese Style

If ever I feel I have slightly over-indulged this is the perfect antidote, a simple and clean way to enjoy produce at its best. You could serve these veg as an accompaniment, but I often prefer to have them just as they are. It's especially satisfying if you are able to pick the veg straight from the garden, sun-warmed and full of goodness.

Serves 2–4

An assortment of seasonal vegetables, e.g.:
  pumpkins or squash, sweet potatoes (peeled),
  carrots (peeled), cauliflower, broccoli, green beans,
  sugar snap peas, asparagus
Flaky sea salt
Good quality olive oil
½ lemon

For the dipping sauce
50ml good quality soy sauce
2 tablespoons mirin
4cm piece of fresh ginger, peeled and finely grated
2 teaspoons maple syrup
½ teaspoon toasted sesame oil

To serve
Small handful of chopped spring onions
2 tablespoons lightly toasted sunflower seeds
2 tablespoons lightly toasted pumpkin seeds
2 tablespoons lightly toasted sesame seeds

Equipment
1 steamer or a 3-tiered bamboo steamer
  that will fit inside a large lidded pot

Once you have chosen your veg, wash them all and cut them into largish bite-size pieces. Arrange them in a single layer with the veg that take longest to cook, for example the pumpkin or squash and sweet potato, together in one basket, broccoli, cauliflower and carrots in another, and quicker-cooking ones like beans and peas in the top basket.

Put your steamer or large pot, with a couple of centimetres of water in the base, over a high heat and bring it to the boil. Don't add too much water or it will rise up through the base of the steamer and boil the veg instead of steaming them.

Place your basket with the longest cooking veg in first. Put the lid on and leave them to steam for about 6–7 minutes, by which time they will be about two-thirds cooked. Now place the second tier in position, cover, and steam for a further 3–4 minutes then place the top tier in position, cover again and steam for 1 minute – this way all the veg should all be ready at the same time: bright yet tender and steamed through. Check by inserting a small sharp knife into the veg – it should slide through easily.

Arrange all the veg on a single plate or tray. Sprinkle with the spring onions and toasted seeds if you wish and take to the table just as it is. Mix together the ingredients for the dipping sauce in a small bowl and serve with the veg.

QUINOA

with a Rainbow of Jewels

I first made this for my friend Ieva on her birthday. It's a beautiful way to present quinoa, the tiny grains and pomegranate seeds really do look like jewels and it's packed with delicious flavours. You can also use this as a base for a hearty stew or casserole, or serve for lunch with some avocado and a green leaf salad.

Serves 6–8
3 small red onions
Good olive oil
½ butternut squash, peeled, cut into 1.5cm squares
700–750g cooked quinoa at room temperature
Seeds from 1 pomegranate
80g parsley, washed and finely chopped
80g mint, washed, leaves picked and finely chopped
juice of 1 lemon
A few fronds of dill, leaves picked
Sea salt and freshly ground black pepper

To serve
Rose petals (optional)

Preheat the oven to 180°C/gas mark 4. Cut the onions in half from top to bottom then peel them, leaving the base intact (you may want to trim off the top, though). Cut each half into 3 wedges – the base will hold the slices together. Put them on a small baking tray, drizzle with olive oil and sprinkle with salt and pepper. Transfer the tray to the oven.

Do the same with the squash on a second tray. Keep an eye on them both: after about 15–20 minutes the red onion should be tender and a little caramelised around the edges. As soon as it's ready, remove the tray. The squash will need a further 10–15 minutes before it's tender and a little coloured at the edges.

When both veg are cooked, put the quinoa in a big serving bowl, then lay the squash and red onion on top, scatter over two-thirds of the pomegranate seeds, the parsley, mint and squeeze over the lemon juice. Drizzle with a generous amount of olive oil. Sprinkle in a good few pinches of sea salt and a few twists of pepper. Using two big spoons, gently toss to mix.

Serve sprinkled with the remaining pomegranate seeds, the dill leaves and rose petals if using.

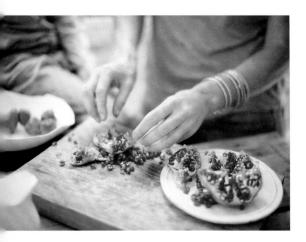

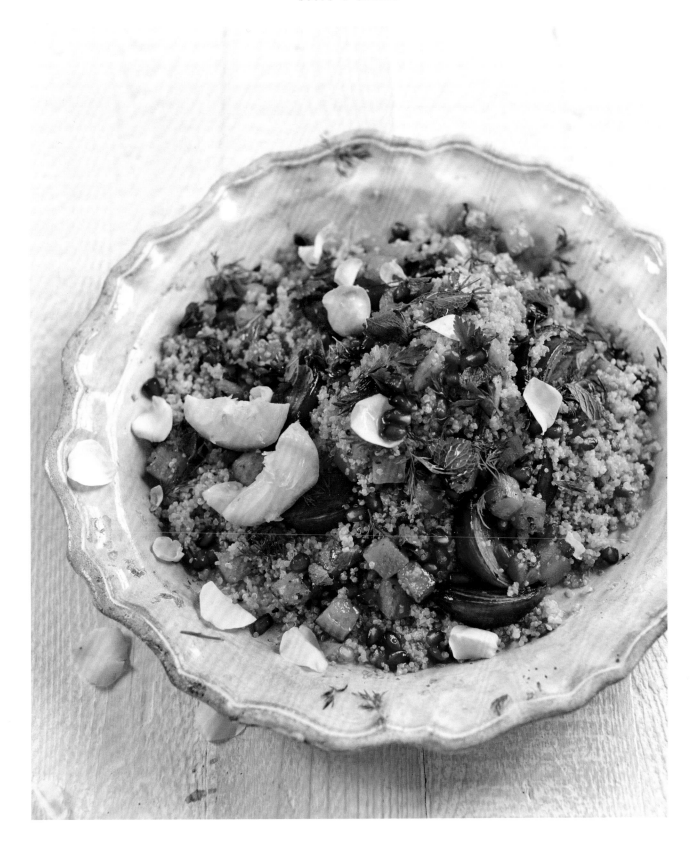

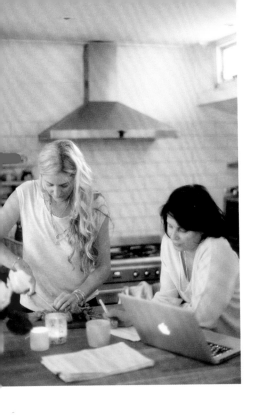

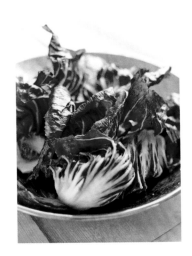

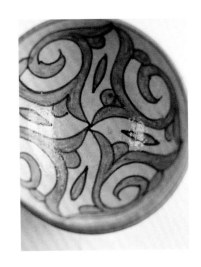

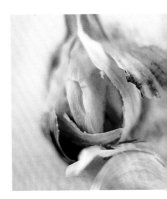

MAIN DISHES

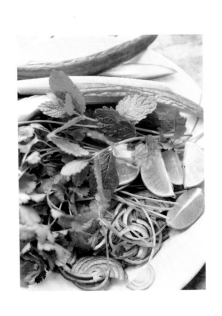

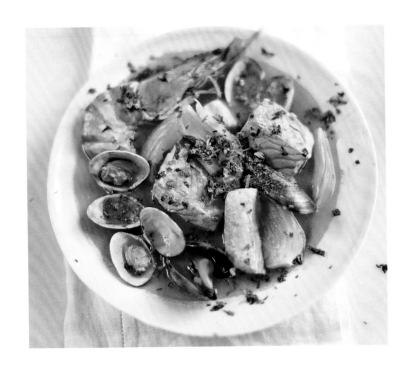

I have based this chapter around ingredients I like to eat for my evening meals, dishes that can be added to or eaten as they are on their own with a simple green salad on the side. There is a cross section – from a simple veg chilli to a sumptuous Mexican feast. All are super healthy and full of goodness, full of immune boosting qualities and good fats. The main meal time of the day for me is dinner. I was bought up in a big family and we always sat down to eat together. This is something I have carried on into my own family with my son. As long as I am not working I will always eat with him. This encourages healthy and positive eating habits and it is a great way to sit and share the day. Sometimes I have the energy to go to town so to speak and other nights dinner can be as simple as an omelette with a green salad. As long as it has some healthy fats and plenty of fibre even a frugal supper can be incredibly nourishing. My taste buds tend to take me around the world and my son loves nothing more than a beautiful curry, freshly made with all good things or the indulgent Mexican feast. For this reason I wanted to include some different bold flavours from around the world, things I cook regularly when I am busy or when I have more time. Either way you will find good nourishment for your body.

MY NOURISH BOWL

two ways

The idea behind a Nourish Bowl is to have something that nourishes all aspects of the self: taste, nutrition and something that nourishes visually. It's about choosing nutrient-dense veggies, healthy fats, quality proteins and some probiotic foods to make a filling meal in a bowl.
It's a great thing to have as a lunch in particular, but could easily work for a delicious dinner. It's endlessly versatile and can be varied to suit what you fancy or what you have in the garden or fridge.
This is more of a guide than a recipe. Here, I show how I may put together my Nourish Bowl, but you can add whatever you like. There are some good things to choose from in the Sides and Mains chapter of this book, so you can build the rest of your Nourish Bowl around things you already have recipes for. For example, if you have a recipe for hummus and you have some chicken or tempeh, that's great: just add some healthy fats and some nutrient-dense veg et voilà!
Whichever ingredients you choose, it should be simple and fun to make, a bit like throwing a beautiful salad together.

For the protein
Tempeh
Fish
Turkey
Chicken
**Eggs, softly boiled with
   runny yolks**
Veg chilli (see page 79)
Cheeses
Lentils
Hummus (see page 107)
Tamari seeds/ toasted seeds
Nuts
Quinoa

For the good fats
**Avocado/guacamole
   (see page 73)**
Cheese
**Cold-pressed oils
   (see page 120)**
Nuts/seeds

Raw and cooked nutrient-dense veg
Beets
Red rose sprouts/ any sprout
Radishes
Globe artichokes
Roast or steamed pumpkin
Tomatoes
Green beans
**Bitter leaves/ rocket/ watercress/
   dandelion/ raddichio/mizuna**

Probiotic foods
Sauerkraut
Kimchi (see page 110)
**Lacto fermented veg
i.e. radishes, cauliflower, carrots**

Arrange what you have chosen and prepared around the bowl. Drizzle with lemon juice and really good quality extra virgin olive oil, and sprinkle with good quality sea salt and freshly cracked pepper.

JAPANESE BROWN RICE BOWL

& Kimchi, two ways

For the protein add either fish or tempeh, a fermented, cooked soya bean product for Indonesia which has more protein and fibre than the more familiar tofu. Brown rice and quinoa are both fantastic for the fibre and micro nutrients they provide.

Serves 6–8
700–750g cooked brown rice or quinoa

For the roasted veg
1 medium pumpkin or butternut squash, halved, seeds removed and sliced into long wedges
Knob of ginger, peeled and grated
1 garlic clove, finely grated
2 teaspoons toasted sesame oil
2 tablespoons tamari, shoyu or other good quality soy sauce
2 tablespoons cold-pressed sunflower oil

For the caramelised sprouts
500g Brussels sprouts, washed and trimmed (or other green veg – beans or broccoli)
3–4 tablespoons cold-pressed sunflower oil
Sea salt and pepper to taste

For the protein
Vegetarian: 1 pack of tempeh, cut into 1.5cm slices and added to the pumpkin when roasting
Fish: 12 small sardines or 4 medium mackerel, cleaned
Olive oil
Juice of ½ lemon
Sea salt and freshly ground black pepper

To serve
2 teaspoons furiyaki or 2 teaspoons toasted black or white sesame seeds
Extra tamari for drizzling on the rice or quinoa
Small bowl of Kimchi (see page 110)
1 lemon, cut into wedges

Preheat the oven to 180°C/gas mark 4. Put the pumpkin on a roasting tray and toss with the other ingredients. If you're following the vegetarian option, add your tempeh to the tray, too.

Roast for 30 minutes or until the pumpkin is tender right through and starting to brown at the edges.

Meanwhile caramelise your Brussels sprouts. Half-fill a medium saucepan with boiling water, place it over a high heat, drop in the sprouts and blanch for about 2 minutes. Remove from the heat and plunge into cold water. Drain, dry the sprouts and cut each one in half.

Set a frying pan over a relatively high heat, add the oil and toss in the sprouts. Cook, stirring every so often, until lovely and caramelised (6–8 minutes). Do keep an eye on them as the sugars in the sprouts mean they can burn easily. Once cooked, remove from the heat and set aside to keep warm.

If you are adding fish to your meal, preheat a griddle pan until smoking hot. Wash the sardines or mackerel, dry them with kitchen paper, toss in a little oil, and place on the hot griddle pan. Cook on both sides until charred; this should take 2–3 minutes on each side for sardines and 5–6 minutes for mackerel; you can always finish them in the oven if it's easier and less smoky. Remove from the heat and squeeze over the lemon juice, and season with a little salt and pepper.

To serve, place the different components into lovely serving bowls and allow people to help themselves.

JAPANESE CHICKEN

This is super and you can also make it using fillets of white fish or salmon as well – just don't cook for so long. It's AMAZING with My Smashed Cucumber Salad (see page 56) and roast pumpkin, brown rice or quinoa – or beetroot quinoa for a super-colourful plate.

Serves 4–6
8–10 chicken thighs, bone in, skin removed

For the marinade
4 fat garlic cloves, finely grated
4cm piece of root ginger, peeled and finely grated
2 teaspoons fermented brown miso
3 tablespoons dark honey
3 tablespoons naturally fermented tamari (Clearspring is a good brand)
½ teaspoon chilli powder (if you can find it togarashi is amazing – omit if feeding children)

To serve
Smashed Cucumber Salad (see page 56).

Wash and dry the chicken thighs. Mix all the marinade ingredients in a large bowl.

Add the chicken and toss the pieces really well to make sure they are well coated. Cover and place in the fridge for several hours or overnight.

Preheat the oven to 180°C/gas mark 4.

Place the chicken pieces in a shallow roasting dish, so that the pieces fit in a single layer quite snugly. Pour over the sauce. Transfer the dish to the oven and roast for 50 minutes, basting every now and then.

Meanwhile, you can prepare the cucumber salad.

The chicken is cooked when all the juices are running clear when poked with the tip of a sharp knife and the meat is starting to fall off the bone.

Serve with brown rice or quinoa.

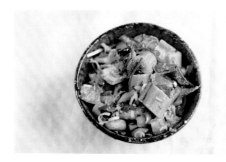

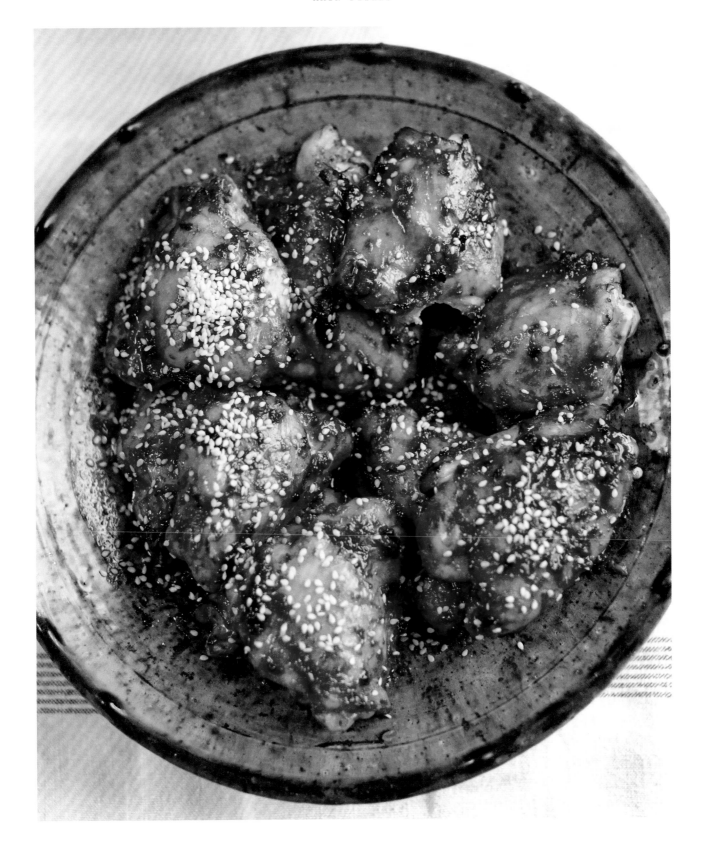

LEMON & SUMAC CHICKEN

with Cherry Tomatoes & Black Olives

This is easy to throw together but it's still full of flavour and colour. My favourite kind of meal... It would be good with Fennel and Blood Orange Salad (see page 54) for a light summery lunch or dinner or with Roast Pumpkin, Golden Beets and Squash Salad (see page 59), for a more nourishing winter meal. Kids and adults both love this and it's a firm favourite in my household.

Serves 4–6
4 free-range whole chicken legs
Handful of good quality black olives
Olive oil
2 teaspoons sumac
Large handful of sweet ripe cherry tomatoes
1 preserved lemon, sliced into thin rounds
Sea salt and freshly cracked or ground black pepper

Preheat the oven to 180°C/gas mark 4.

Wash and dry the chicken pieces and place in a roasting dish. Scatter the black olives on top, and drizzle with olive oil. Sprinkle with the sumac and some salt and black pepper.

Transfer the dish to the middle rack of the oven and cook for 30 minutes. Top with the cherry tomatoes and lemon slices then cook for a further 20–30 minutes – you want the tomatoes bursting, the lemons a little charred and the meat falling off the bone.

Serve while hot and fresh from the oven. I love to eat this chicken dish with a beautiful bitter raddichio salad.

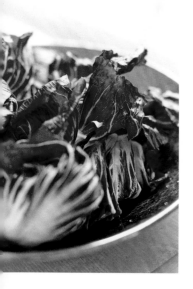

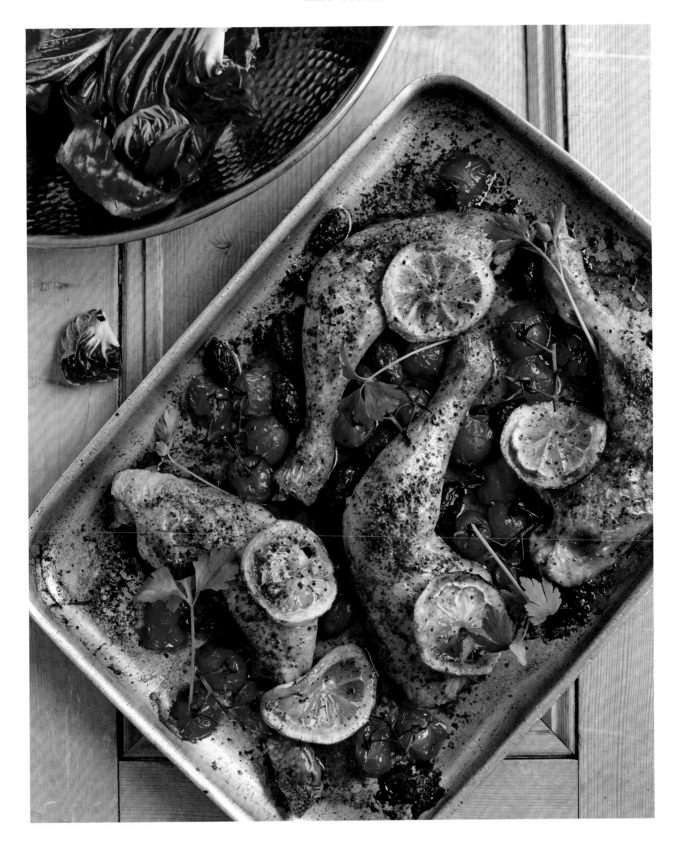

MEXICAN FEAST

Mexican Feast serves 4-6

To serve
2 packs of fresh corn tortillas
200ml soured cream

Prepare the chicken first then, whilst it's marinating, prepare the other recipes. When you are ready to eat, toast your corn tortillas in a hot pan, allowing 30 seconds per side, then pile them onto a plate and cover with a tea towel as you go to keep them warm.

Simply lay everything onto the table and make up tortillas with different combinations each time as and how you like. Serve with the corn alongside and top your tortillas with either soured cream or slices of pickled red onion or both! Enjoy.

REFRIED BEANS WITH FETA

Olive oil
1 large onion, finely diced
1 garlic clove, finely chopped
1 x 400g tin black pinto beans and their liquid
1 teaspoon chipotle chilli powder, plus a little extra
Sea salt and freshly ground black pepper
100g feta

Heat a little oil in a medium saucepan, add the onion and sauté for about 5 minutes, then add the garlic and beans, liquid and all. Simmer gently for about 20 minutes. Add the chipotle powder and simmer for a further 5 minutes. If the beans are getting too dry, add a little water, as they will thicken up as they cool – don't make them too liquid, though. Remove from the heat, scoop into a bowl and crumble over the feta. Sprinkle with a little extra chipotle powder.

GUACAMOLE

6 ripe avocados, halved, pits removed
Zest and juice of 1 lemon
2 limes, zest of 1 and juice of both
1 medium red onion, finely diced
2 garlic cloves, finely grated
Small bunch of coriander, roughly chopped, plus extra sprigs to serve
8 tablespoons cold-pressed olive oil, plus extra to drizzle
Sea salt and freshly ground pepper.

Scoop the flesh of the avocados into a medium bowl and mash with a fork. Squeeze over the lemon and lime juice, mix, then add all the other ingredients. Check the seasoning, adding a little salt and pepper to taste. Scrape into a lovely serving bowl, drizzle with a little olive oil and garnish with a few sprigs of coriander.

CHARGRILLED SWEETCORN WITH SMOKED PAPRIKA & SALT

4 sweetcorn on the cob, husks removed and each cob cut into 3
2 tablespoons cold-pressed sunflower oil
1 teaspoon smoked paprika
1 teaspoon sea salt and a few twists of black pepper

Bring a medium pan of water to the boil, drop in the sweetcorn, simmer gently with the lid on for about 10 minutes; drain, dry and set aside.

Bring a griddle pan to smoking point. While the pan is heating, drizzle the oil over the sweetcorn and then place them carefully onto the hot griddle, moving every now and then to char on all sides – this should take 2–3 minutes.

Remove from the pan and sprinkle with the salt and smoked paprika. Pile the sweetcorn high onto a beautiful plate.

PICKLED RED ONIONS

2 teaspoons black peppercorns
8 whole allspice berries
2 cloves
1 level teaspoon oregano
1 medium red onion, peeled, halved and sliced into thin half moons
¾ teaspoon sea salt
50ml apple cider vinegar
3 juicy limes, squeezed

First grind the peppercorns, allspice, cloves and oregano to a coarse powder using a pestle and mortar or a spice grinder.

Put the sliced onion into a medium bowl, add the spice mix and massage it into the onion, then add salt, vinegar and lime juice. Mix everything really well.

Transfer the mix to tall narrow jar with a tightly fitting lid. Leave it marinate for 24 hours, giving the jar an occasional shake, before using. These pickled onions will keep in the fridge for up to a week.

PICO DE GALLO

300g mix of heritage and cherry tomatoes
1 medium red chilli, finely diced
1 medium green chilli, finely diced
1 small red onion, finely diced
1 garlic clove, finely grated
Juice of 1 lime
Zest and juice of ½ lemon
Small bunch of coriander, washed, drained and roughly chopped

Chop all the tomatoes into small pieces – either into halves or quarters, depending on size. Put them in a bowl along with all the other ingredients and mix thoroughly. Transfer to a serving bowl and keep cool until ready to use.

MY MEXICAN FRESH SALAD

1 red onion, peeled, halved lengthways and sliced into thin half moons
1 cucumber, washed and cut into finger-size pieces
Bunch of coriander, washed and drained
2 limes, each cut into 8 wedges

Arrange all the ingredients on a beautiful plate.

SHREDDED CHICKEN THIGHS MARINATED WITH GINGER & CHILLI

8 chicken thighs, skins removed
4 dried guajillo chillies, wiped clean, destemmed, slit open, deseeded and deveined
2cm piece of ginger, peeled
2 garlic cloves
1 teaspoon ground cumin
1½ teaspoons salt
150ml cold-pressed olive oil

Place the chicken thighs in a large bowl. Soak the dried chillies in warm water for 30 minutes. Drain and put in a food processor with the ginger, garlic, cumin, salt and olive oil. Add 100ml of water and blitz until smooth. Pour the marinade over the chicken and massage gently. Cover the bowl for at least 4 hours or overnight to marinate.

Preheat the oven to 180°C/gas mark 4. Transfer the chicken and all the marinade into an ovenproof dish and roast gently for about 1 hour, or until the meat really starts to fall off the bone.

Remove from the oven and carefully shred all the chicken off the bone in large flakes using two forks. Place the shredded chicken into a lovely serving bowl for the feast.

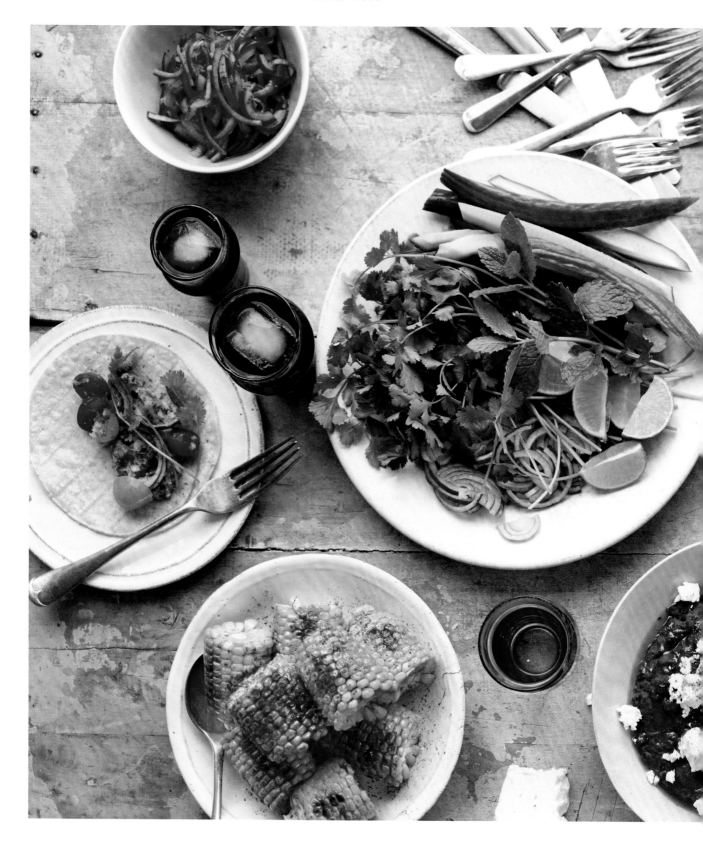

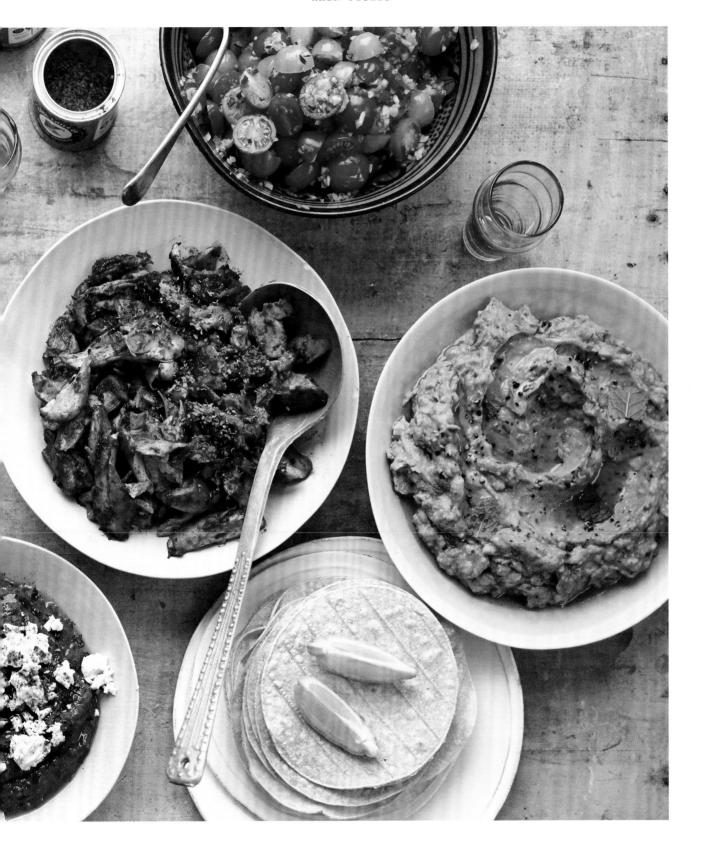

A PERFECTLY COOKED PIECE OF FISH

Serves 1
1 fillet of fish with skin on or off, roughly 230g per person (salmon, sea bass, pollock, cod, snapper, hake, red mullet)
Sea salt and pepper
Olive oil or ghee or grape-seed oil
A knob of butter
½ lemon

Get a heavy-bottomed steel pan very hot over a medium to high heat for several minutes before you start cooking. A nonstick pan won't get the skin really brown and golden.

First wash the fillet, then dry it well with a paper towel to make the skin crisp. Season both sides with sea salt and pepper.

Coat a hot pan with a little oil, something with a high smoke point like ghee or grape-seed is great. Allow the oil to heat and, when it starts to smoke, quickly add your fish, skin side down. The proteins will immediately react and the fillet will contract and curve upwards. Take a flexible spatula and press the entire fillet gently back down and hold for a few seconds to ensure even cooking and crispy skin all over.

Flip near the end of cooking. Let the fish cook, don't mess with it too much, just let it go. When you can see a lovely golden brown colour on the edge of the skin, and the edges of the fish are turning an opaque colour, carefully and gently use a spatula to life up the fillet and turn it over. The fish is delicate, so flip it carefully so it doesn't all break up. At this point it's about 70 per cent cooked, so it will only need another couple of minutes on the next side.

You can add a knob of butter at this point for flavour if you like and baste the fish while it finishes cooking. Remove from the pan and serve.

BAKED POLLOCK

with Ginger, Tomatoes & Pine Nuts

This is one of those wonderful recipes that look great, tastes amazing and yet is so easy to make. It's great with a big green salad, or Puy Lentils with Wilted Spinach (see page 53). It's a great summery dish.

Serves 4
4 medium fillets of pollock (roughly 180g each)

For the marinade
Small handful of basil leaves, torn
1 medium red chilli, deseeded and finely sliced
3 tablespoons olive oil
Generous handful of cherry tomatoes
Generous pinch of sea salt flakes
30ml lemon juice
30ml water
2cm piece of ginger, peeled and finely grated
1 garlic clove, finely grated
150g pine nuts

To serve
10 mint leaves torn
½ red chilli, deseeded and sliced into thin circles
Small handful of torn basil leaves

Put the fish fillets in a roasting dish just big enough to hold them comfortably without being too cramped.

Mix the ingredients for the fish marinade and rub over the fillets, cover and leave to marinate for 1 hour.

Preheat the oven to 180°C/gas mark 4. Transfer the marinated fish to the middle rack of the oven and cook for 12–15 minutes, depending on the size of the fillets. Once cooked, remove from the oven and allow to sit for a further 2 minutes.

Sprinkle with torn mint leaves, extra chilli and basil. Serve immediately.

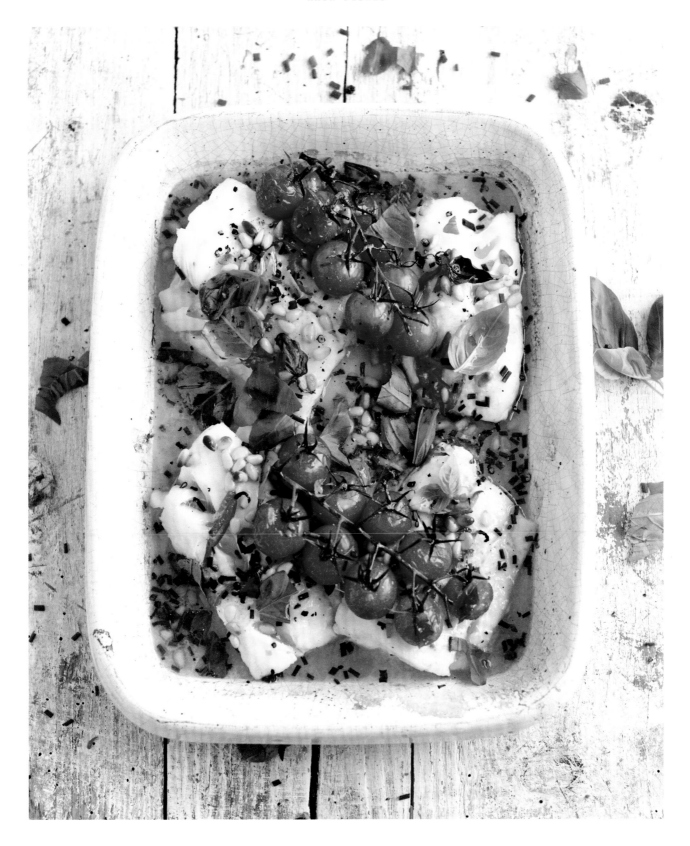

SEAFOOD & FENNEL STEW

with Tarragon Gremolata

This is a winning combination of Mediterranean flavours – seafood, fennel, tomatoes, garlic and preserved lemon – and the tarragon gremolata really makes the dish sing. I will happily eat this stew on its own, but it would also be rather good served on a bed of quinoa.

Serves 6
Good drizzle olive oil
3 large garlic cloves, finely sliced
3 fennel bulbs, trimmed and cut into wedges, fronds reserved for garnish
650ml fish stock
½ medium preserved lemon, chopped into 4
8 large vine tomatoes, quartered
1 tablespoon sweet paprika
Good pinch of saffron
Small handful of chopped flatleaf parsley
2 fillets of salmon, (250g) skin removed, cut into 3
2 fillets of cod or other white fish, (250g) skin removed, cut into 3
12 mussels
24 clams
6 tiger prawns (the really big ones)
Sea salt and freshly ground black pepper

To serve
Tarragon Gremolata (see page 106)

Put the olive oil and garlic in a large, heavy-based pan or stock pot and cook over a medium-low heat for 2 minutes. Add the fennel wedges and cook for a further 3–4 minutes.

Stir in the stock and the preserved lemon, bring to the boil and then cover and reduce the heat to a gentle simmer and cook for 10 minutes. Add the tomatoes, spices and the parsley. Cook for a further 5 minutes.

Add the pieces of fish, the seafood and up to 200ml water – enough to ensure the liquid in the pan covers the fish.

Put a lid on the pan and turn up the heat to a rolling boil. Cook for 3-4 minutes, or until the shellfish has opened and the prawns are pink.

Using a slotted spoon, remove the shellfish and fish from the stew and allow continue to cook, uncovered, for 4–5 minutes until the soup liquid has reduced and slightly thickened.

Taste for seasoning and add salt and pepper if required. Return the shellfish and fish to the pan for a minute or two. Serve hot, sprinkled with the tarragon gremolata.

My mum's

VEG CHILLI

This is a super easy chilli that lasts really well. It's packed full of protein and flavour. Kids love it, as do adults. I like to make big batches and keep it in the fridge, so it's easy to knock up a great dinner or lunch in 5 minutes. It's perfect after a strenuous day or a long exercise session. My favourite way of eating it is with crème fraîche and coriander.

Serves 4–6

4 garlic cloves
4 tablespoons cold-pressed sunflower oil, raw coconut
   oil or you can use ghee
1 large yellow onion, finely diced
1 large carrot, peeled and cut into 1cm dice
1 red pepper, halved, deseeded and ribs removed, cut
   into 1cm dice
½ teaspoon mild chilli powder
1 teaspoon cumin
2 teaspoons chipotle in adobo sauce (or chipotle
   powder can be used)
800g passata (preferably from a glass jar)
110g puy lentils, rinsed
1 x 400g tin black beans, rinsed and drained (or 400g
   fresh black beans after soaking and cooking)
1 x 400g tin kidney beans rinsed and drained
   (same as above)
4 tablespoons tomato paste
Hearty pinch of sea salt and plenty of freshly cracked
   or ground black pepper
Small bunch of fresh coriander,
   washed and finely chopped

To serve
Fresh soured cream or crème fraîche
Fresh coriander leaves
Chilli powder or extra chipotle

Start by mincing or chopping your garlic really finely and allow it to sit for 10 minutes while you prepare the rest of the veg.

Heat the oil in a large saucepan or stock pot over a high heat. Add the onion, carrot, pepper, garlic, chilli powder and cumin, along with a hearty pinch of salt. When everything is hot and cooking nicely, turn the heat down a little and continue to sweat all the veg for about 10–15 minutes. You want them softened, sweet and not colouring too much. After 15 minutes stir in the chipotle.

At this point, turn the heat back up, add the plum tomatoes (or homemade bottled tomatoes as my mum would), and be sure to tip in all the juices too.
Bring to the boil.

To help the tomatoes break up a bit, gently crush them with a wooden spoon or spatula. Reduce the heat and allow the veg to simmer for 25 minutes.

Throw in your rinsed lentils and beans and add one can of water to the pot, along with the tomato paste. Bring to the boil, reduce the heat and simmer for 1 hour 20 minutes, adding a touch more water if it dries out too much. After it's cooked, allow to settle and cool a bit. Serve while hot with some lovely sour cream and coriander.

SPRING COURGETTI

with Rocket Flowers

Making spaghetti from courgettes couldn't be easier, but you do need a spiraliser or special peeler - they are easy to find on line or in kitchen shops. I have teamed my courgetti here with spring peas and kale pesto and rocket flowers. The rocket flowers are spicy and nutty; if you can't find the flowers you can just use rocket leaves. This is really light and delicious yet a very nutrient dense dish which will certainly give you a spring in your step. As this dish is raw it's great for late spring or early summer when lighter and more refreshing meals are the order of the day.

Serves 2
2 courgettes, spiralised

For the kale pesto
85g cashew nuts, lightly toasted
85g parmesan, coarsely grated
3 garlic cloves
75ml extra virgin olive oil
85g kale, leafy part only, not the inner stalk
a good squeeze of lemon

To serve
Big drizzle extra virgin, cold-pressed olive oil
Torn basil leaves
Torn mint leaves
A handful of fresh podded peas or lightly blanched frozen peas
Rocket flowers or a handful of rocket leaves
Shavings of parmesean
Sea salt and freshly cracked black pepper

Place everything for the pesto into a blender and blitz until you have a rough sauce, adding a little bit more lemon juice or parmesan to taste if it needs more balance, and season to taste.

Place your courgetti into a lovely big serving bowl, top with the kale pesto and the olive oil and toss to coat the courgetti. Strew with torn basil leaves, mint leaves, peas, rocket leaves or flowers, shavings of parmesean and a few twists of pepper.

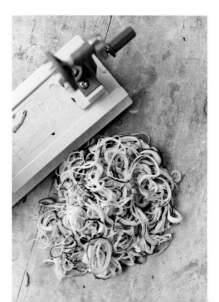

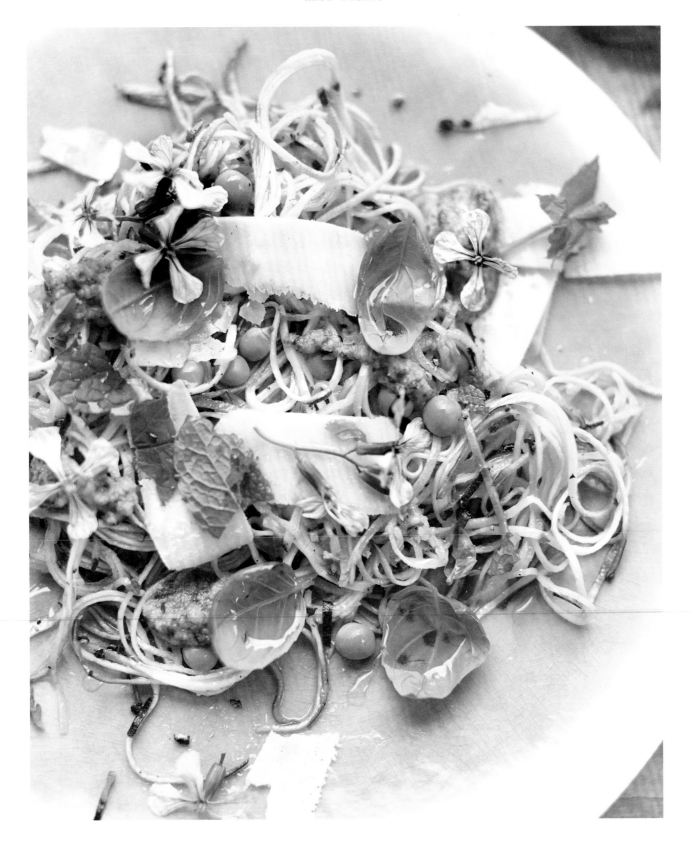

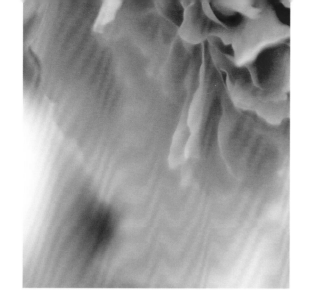

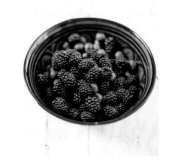

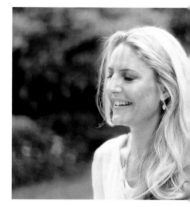

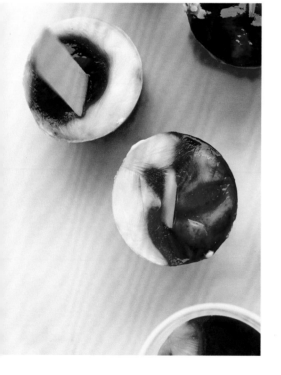

SWEET TOOTH

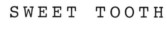

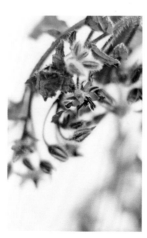

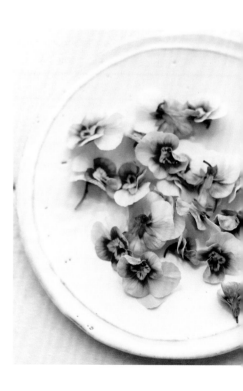

As you may know, I have a bit of a sweet tooth. My last book was a healthy baking book and I have included in this chapter some more delightful things that happen in my kitchen on a regular basis. Everything from a 3-layered celebration cake to healthy ice cream, decadent but super-nourishing and totally good for you.

There are also some great snack ideas for those moments when we need a little pick up, when reserves are low. If you're like me and need to keep your energy levels up, and find it hard to make wise choices when sugar levels are low then it's not fair to rely on will power alone.

I would strongly recommend having a few things on hand in jars ready to eat when you need a quick pick-me-up. I always have soaked almonds in the fridge and a jar of grain-free granola on my shelf; it's perfect as a little snack.

My son loves ice cream, so I have come up with healthy ideas for ices that adults love too. Always have some frozen bananas and berries in your freezer ready to go. Then you can build on those flavours with other things that are in season or in your store cupboard. I am sure you will find plenty of inspiration in these next few pages for healthy snacks and treats.

CHIA PUDDING

with Apple Compôte, Fresh Raspberries and Pistachios

This pudding is full of flavour, with healthy fats and omega oils from the chia seeds and coconut milk. Healthy fats help to stabilize metabolism. Chia pudding is so easy to make and hits the spot when you need a bit of a treat. I love to make extra chia pudding to keep in the fridge so that I can add some fresh fruit and coconut yoghurt whenever I need a little pick me up or for my son's afternoon tea. It will keep well there for up to a week.

Serves 2
340ml of your favourite milk, heated
4 tablespoons chia seeds
1 large bramley apple,
  peeled, cored and cut into
  3cm pieces
1–2 teaspoons raw date syrup
  or raw honey
¼ pod of vanilla, seeds scraped out
50g chopped pistachios
Borage flowers (optional)

Start by pouring the hot milk into a bowl, add the chia seeds and stir. Allow to sit for 5 minutes, then stir briskly again to break up any lumps. Stir again after a further 5 minutes, cover and allow to soak for several hours or overnight. This allows the breakdown of any anti nutrients (see note below), and makes the soaked seeds a lot more digestible and nutritious.

While your seeds are soaking, you can make the simple apple compôte. Place the apple in a small saucepan with a couple of tablespoons of water and the vanilla seeds, place over a medium heat with a tightly fitting lid. When it starts to bubble and steam, stir after a minute or two. It should take about 10 minutes to cook and break down. I like it still with some texture, not totally puréed. When it's softened, add the honey or date syrup to taste. At this point reheat your chia pudding by placing it in a small saucepan with a tablespoon or 2 of water and warm through.

Scoop the pudding into 2 bowls, top with the apple compôte and a sprinkling of chopped pistachios or any other favourite nut. Toasted chopped almonds are delicious. If you have any borage flowers they look beautiful sprinkled over. Serve while warm.

* Anti nutrients are natural or synthetic compounds that interfere with the absorption of nutrients. They are found in the skins or coating of most seeds/nuts and grains. To neutralise the anti nutrients you can soak your seeds/nuts/grains for several hours or overnight. Times vary depending on what you are soaking.

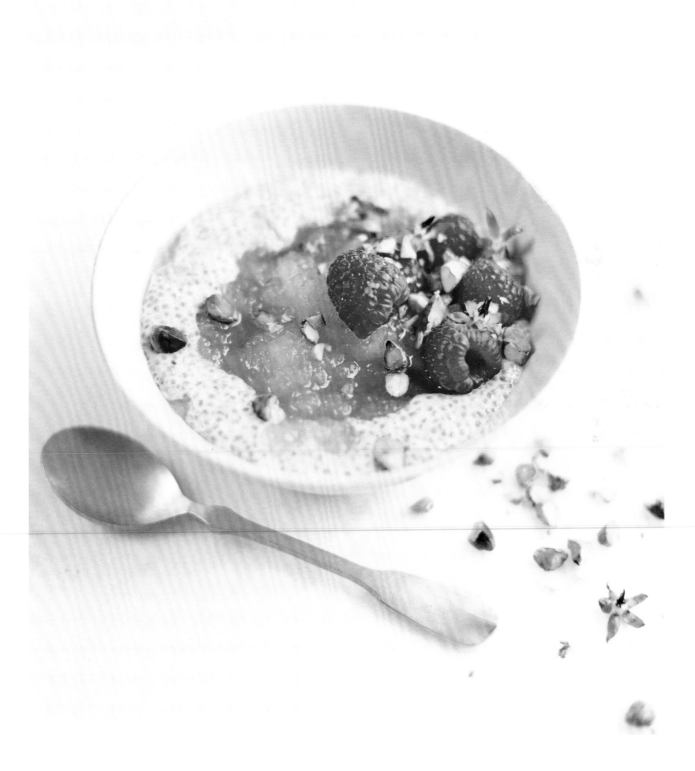

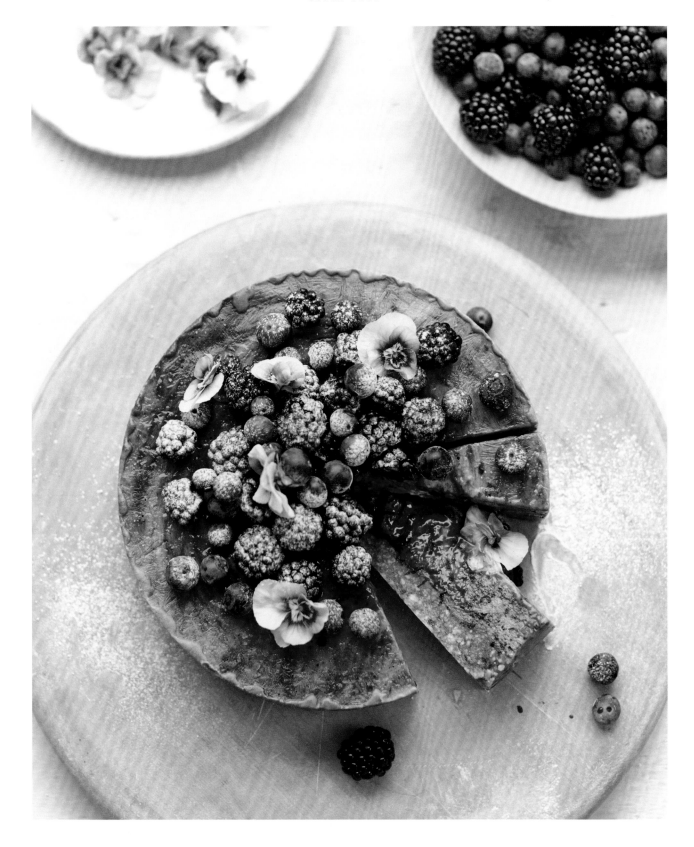

BLACKBERRY & ROSE CHEESECAKE

with Flowers

This is a super fresh and decadent frozen cheescake, a bit like an ice cream cake but healthy for you. It's easy to put together and really refreshing on a hot summer's evening for an outside dinner party. The crust is wonderfully chewy and nutty and the yoghurt topping is everything it should be, fruity and fragrant and creamy.

Serves 12

For the crust
300g blanched almonds
50g sunflower seeds
12 fresh medjool dates, pitted
Zest of ½ lemon
2 tablespoons raw coconut oil
Hearty pinch of sea salt

For the filling
200g blackberries
100g blueberries
Juice of ½ lemon
120ml raw honey
500g Greek yoghurt or
    thick coconut yoghurt
1 teaspoon rosewater

For the topping
250g blackberries
100g blueberries

Flowers to decorate, preferably purple ones
    (eg sweet peas, rose petals, lavender,
    cornflowers, violas)

Preheat the oven to 180°C/gas mark 4. Spread the almonds and sunflower seeds on a baking tray and roast in the oven for about 6–8 minutes, or until they are starting to colour a little and smell nutty. Remove from the oven and allow to cool a little.

Tip the nuts into a food processor and blitz just enough to chop them but do not let them become powdered. Add the dates, lemon zest, coconut oil and a pinch of salt and blitz again until the mix comes together and you have a lovely looking sticky mixture.

Scrape the mixture into a 20cm nonstick, loose-based cake tin and press it flat, but don't squash. Place in the fridge to chill and set.

Purée the blackberries and blueberries in the food processor along with the lemon juice and honey. Scrape the mix into a large bowl and add the yoghurt. Fold everything together until completely combined.

Spoon the topping over the chilled base and smooth it evenly using the back of a spoon. Put in the freezer and leave it to set for at least 3–4 hours. It needs to be frozen almost completely. The very middle is nice if it still has a bit of a wobble, but as it has no gelatin it will not hold if it's not frozen. If you have frozen it overnight, move it to the fridge for half an hour before serving.

When you are ready to serve, simply bring the cheesecake out of the freezer (or fridge) and carefully unmould from the tin. Decorate with the extra berries and lots of petals.

A DECADENT CHOCOLOLATE MOUSSE

with Raspberry, Rose Compôte & Pistachios

You won't believe how simple it is to make this mousse, how delicious it tastes and how amazingly good for you it is. Chocolate has a natural affinity for tart raspberries and the delicate floral notes of rosewater. The pistachios add colour and a pleasing crunch.

Serves 2–3

For the mousse
80ml raw honey or maple syrup
2 ripe avocadoes
1 ripe banana
Seeds from ½ vanilla pod
30g raw cacao powder

For the compôte
300g fresh raspberries
Juice of ½ lemon
2 tablespoons maple syrup or honey
½ teaspoon rosewater

To serve
100g pistachios, roughly chopped
Rose petals (must be unsprayed), to decorate

To make the mousse, simply put all the ingredients into a powerful blender and blitz until you have a smooth mousse. If you want a lighter consistency add a small splash of coconut water. Scrape into a serving bowl or individual bowls and put in the fridge to set, roughly 20 minutes.

Meanwhile, macerate your berries. Put the raspberries into a bowl, squeeze over the lemon juice and pour in the syrup and rosewater. Mix well with a spoon, ever so lightly crushing the berries. Set aside for 10–15 minutes to macerate.

When the mousse is set and the berries are ready, simply spoon the berries over the mousse, top with chopped pistachios and scatter a few petals. A heavenly pudding – it's a feast for the eyes as well as the taste buds. Dust with more cacao powder if you like.

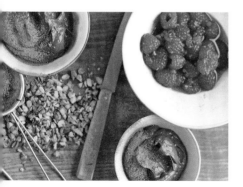

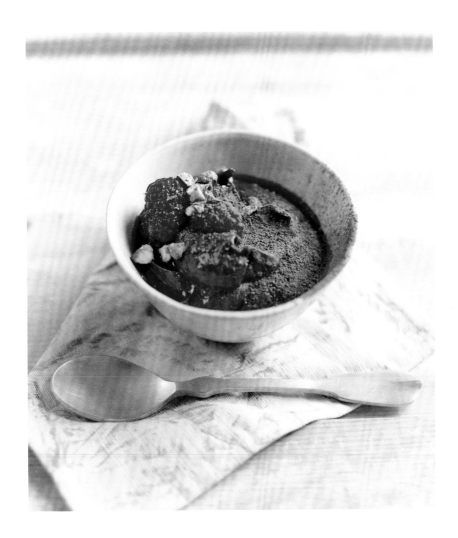

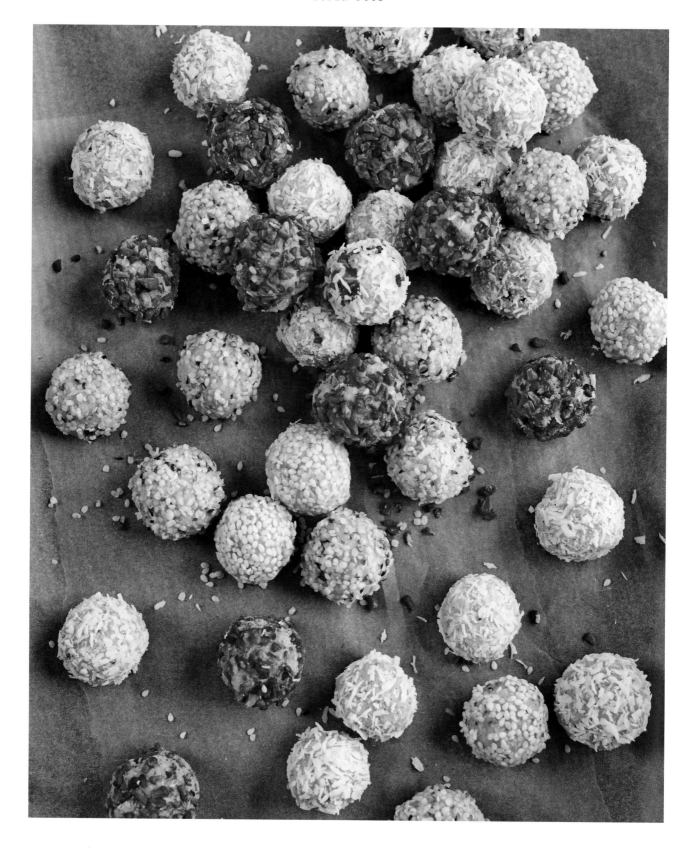

COCONUT & APRICOT
BLISS BALLS

These wonderfully delicious little balls are perfect as a snack for packed lunches or afternoon tea, or any time for that matter. They last really well in the fridge, so once you have made a big batch they can be kept in the fridge for when you need them. They are light and moist and can be coated with different things, which is great – you can coat some with nuts and some with seeds, and sometimes I like to coat some with freeze-dried berries, then you have some for all taste buds.

Makes approx 40 balls
1 medium, mature coconut
200g sulphur-free dried apricots, plus 5 extra
**Small handful of pistachio or cashew nuts,
 roughly chopped**
1 generous tablespoon raw honey

To coat, use a few tablespoons of any of the following
Sesame seeds
Shelled hemp seeds
Freeze-dried raspberries
Desiccated coconut

First soak the dried apricots (except for the 5 extra) for 6–8 hours.

Make two holes in the coconut and drain the liquid through a fine sieve to catch any bits. Reserve the liquid for later use.

Break the shell open, scoop out the coconut flesh and give it a quick rinse to wash off any bits of shell. Cut the coconut flesh into pieces and put through a juicer.

Drain the soaked apricots and mix with the coconut pulp. Blitz with a stick blender or in a food processor (you could do this by hand if you mash and chop the soaked fruit really finely or use a large mortar and pestle). If the mix is too dry, spoon in a little reserved coconut water to bring it all together. Roughly chop the 5 extra apricots and add, together with the chopped nuts, to the mixture.

Use your hands to roll the mixture into small balls and then roll each one in your chosen coating. Place on a large tray or plate and transfer to the fridge to set.

These balls keep well in a cool place. Keep in the fridge until you're going to eat them.

RASPBERRY & ROSE
CUPCAKES

Sometimes life calls for something sweet, pretty and delicious to mark an occasion. These are just the thing. Whether it's an afternoon tea or a picnic, they will impress. Sometimes I leave them un-iced and have them as breakfast muffins. As they are full of nuts, fibre and natural sweetening, they are a great way to kick start the day. The cream topping doesn't last long, so they are best eaten soon after icing them.

Makes 18
220g ground almonds
100g desiccated coconut
1 large ripe banana, mashed
3 free-range eggs
4 tablespoons melted coconut oil, butter or ghee
125ml kefir (or plain natural yoghurt, or full-fat coconut milk well blended)
10 medjool dates, pitted
1½ teaspoons baking powder (you can omit the baking powder but be prepared for a denser cupcake)
Seeds from ½ vanilla pod
1 teaspoon rosewater
Pinch of sea salt
2 handfuls of fresh raspberries (red or white)

For the cream
1 Cashew Cream (see page 119), plus a handful of fresh raspberries
or
2 Light Coconut Cream with Vanilla (see page 118), plus a handful of fresh raspberries
or
1 Freshly Whipped Cream (see page 118), plus a handful of fresh raspberries

To serve
Rose petals
Small handful of pistachio nuts or almonds, roughly chopped

Preheat the oven to 200°C/gas mark 6. Line 18 cupcake moulds with cases or baking paper.

Put all the ingredients for the cupcakes except the raspberries into a food processor and blitz until well combined. Scrape the mixture into a bowl. (If you don't have a food processor, mash the bananas and dates to a soft mush then add the rest of the ingredients except for the berries and beat with a wooden spoon until throughly combined.) Add the raspberries and gently stir through, then spoon the mixture into the prepared cases. Bake for 10–12 minutes then remove from the oven and transfer to a wire rack to cool.

Meanwhile, prepare your chosen cream and push the raspberries through a sieve to remove the seeds. Fold the pulp and juices through the cream so that you have a lovely marbled effect.

Place dollops of cream on top of the cupcakes and decorate with fresh petals and chopped nuts.

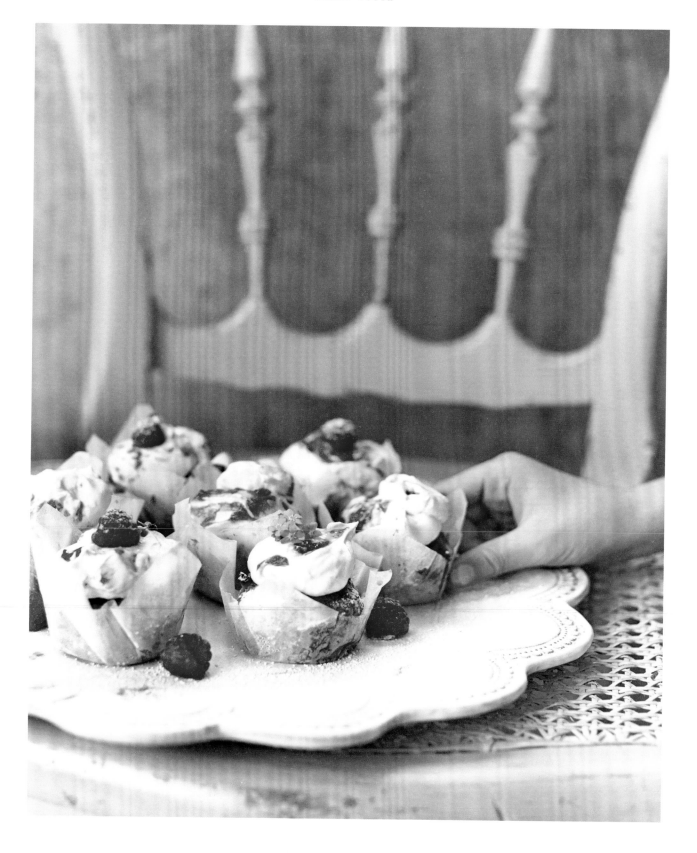

BAKED FIGS & STRAWBERRIES

with Honey, Vanilla & Toasted Almonds

Baked figs and strawberries are a match made in heaven, sweet and decadent. Eat as a pudding or for breakfast with some natural, unsweetened yoghurt to balance the sweet. This is best made in mid to late summer, when the figs are luscious and ripe and the end of the season's strawberries are full of flavour and bursting with sweetness. The almonds add crunch and texture. You can also serve this with Light Coconut Cream (see page 118) if you're not eating dairy.

Serves 6

600g perfectly ripe figs, stalks removed
100g cold butter (or raw cold coconut oil)
250g in-season, smallish strawberries, hulled
150g raw or local honey, light honey is best
1 lemon, zested and juice of half (can use an orange
    as a variation)
1 vanilla pod, seeds scraped out (or 1 teaspoon of
    vanilla essence)
100g flaked almonds

Preheat the oven to 180°C/gas mark 4.

Cut a cross in the top of each fig, then place them into a baking dish that will accommodate them all in a single layer, with a little extra room for the berries. Put a small knob of butter into the top of each fig, scatter over the strawberries. Drizzle the whole thing with the honey, squeeze over the lemon juice, dot on the vanilla seeds and lastly sprinkle over the flaked almonds.

Bake in the oven until the figs are just collapsing, about 10-15 minutes. Take the dish out of the oven and sprinkle with the lemon zest. Serve hot or warm with your favourite yoghurt or cream.

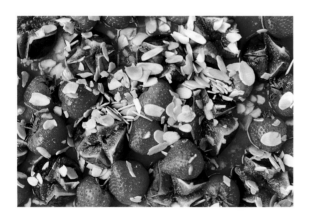

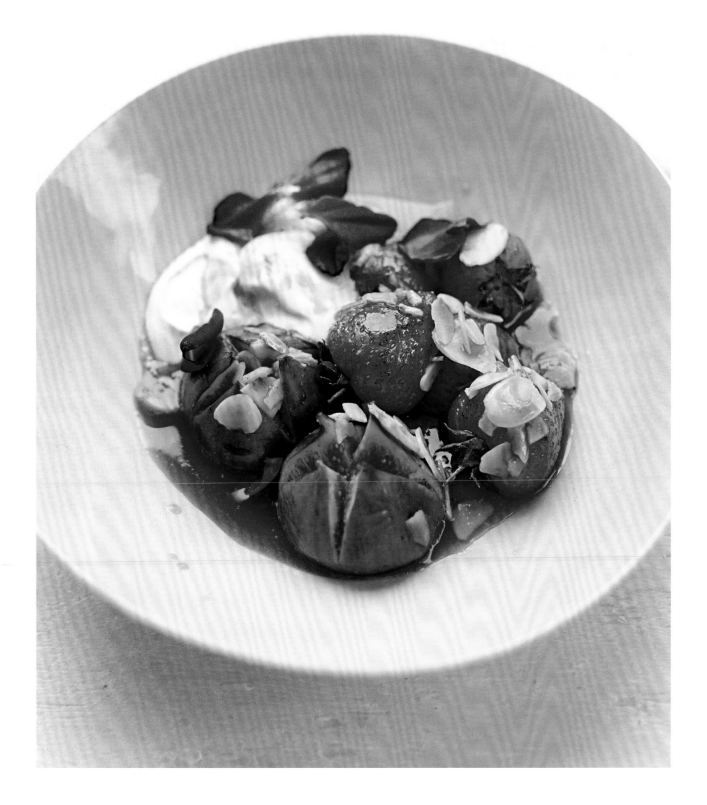

SPICED CHOCOLATE &
SWEET POTATO BROWNIES

*These gluten-free brownies can be eaten just as they are for a delicious afternoon tea
or snack or they can be plated for a special dessert and served with a spoonful of crème
fraîche, a dusting of raw cacao powder and perhaps a few fresh raspberries.*

Makes 16
3 medium sweet potatoes
12 fresh medjool dates, pitted
70g ground almonds
75g buckwheat flour
3 tablespoons raw cacao nibs
4 tablespoons raw cacao
3 tablespoons honey
Zest of 1 orange
½ teaspoon ground cinnamon

To serve
A dusting of raw cacao powder

Preheat the oven to 180°C/gas mark 4 and line a 10 x
20cm brownie tin or baking dish.

Peel your sweet potatoes, put them into a steamer and
steam for about 18–20 minutes or until completely soft.
Remove them from the steamer and transfer to a food
processor along with the pitted dates and blend.

Mix the remaining ingredients in a large bowl, then add
the sweet potato and date mixture to the bowl and fold
everything together.

Spoon the mixture into the lined tin and cook for about
20 minutes. Remove from the oven and allow to cool
a little before dusting with raw cacao powder, cutting
and serving.

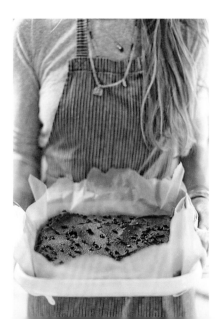

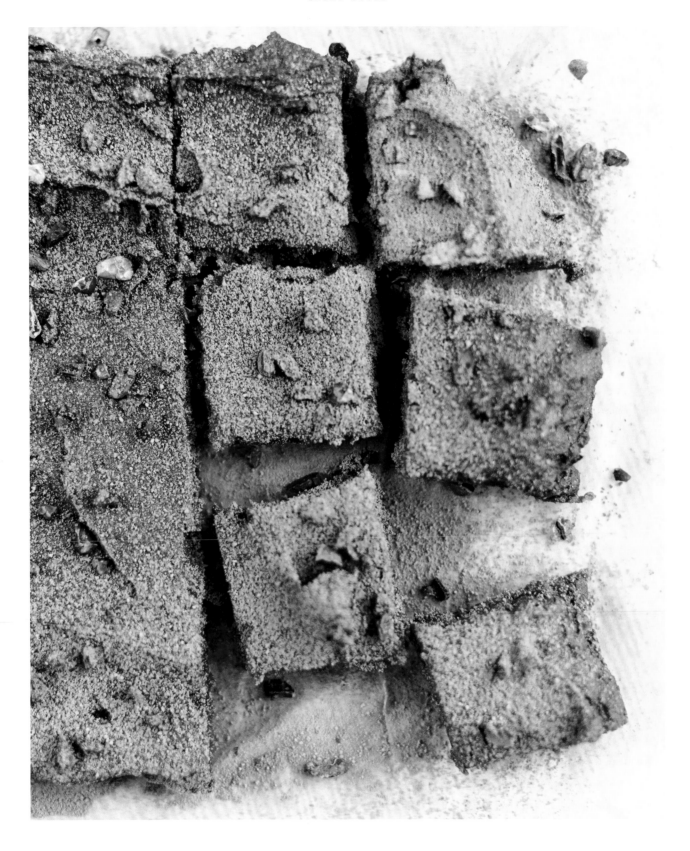

BLACKCURRANT & ROSE COCONUT ICE CREAM

Blackcurrants have quite an intense flavor, so this one is more for the adults. Unless your child likes slightly sour, tart flavours....some do! The rose goes beautifully with the blackcurrants, I tend to like my currants quite tart but if you like them sweeter, just add a bit more honey. These little black berries have gone a bit out of fashion but I think they are marvellous things, full of vitamin C and such a rich, deep purple colour, which contrasts so beautifully with pink rose petals and the emerald green of the pistachio.

Serves 3-4

120g blackcurrants, frozen
60g blackberries, frozen
60g blueberries, frozen
200ml coconut milk, full fat
2 tablespoons raw honey
1 teaspoon rose water

To serve
Small dark pink rose petals
Handful of pistachios, finely chopped

Place all the ingredients into a food processor and blitz until you have a soft serve ice cream. Scoop into bowls, top with rose petals and chopped pistachios and serve immediately.

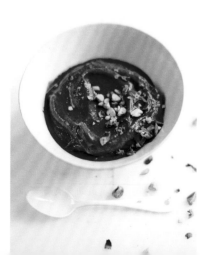

BANANA & RAW CACAO ICE

with Pomegranates & Cacao Nibs

This is a really nourishing and decadent treat. The cacao nibs and pomegranate seeds add a lovely contrasting crunch to its super-creamy texture. The raw cacao powder and nibs are quite bitter, which is how I love my chocolate.

Serves 2–4

4 ripe bananas, sliced into thin rounds
2 tablespoons raw cacao powder
125ml unsweetened almond milk
2 tablespoons maple syrup

To serve
Seeds from 1 pomegranate
2 tablespoons raw cacao nibs

First put your banana slices in a large ziplock bag in the freezer. Lay the bag flat so that the banana slices don't freeze in one big clump; I usually leave mine in the freezer overnight but they will only take a few hours.

When the slices are thoroughly frozen, put them into a food processor or high speed blender with the cacao powder, almond milk and syrup and blitz for 1–2 minutes, scraping down the sides as necessary. The bananas will thaw a little, melting beautifully into the other components to make that delicious velvety-smooth ice cream texture.

Once you have the right consistency, scrape the ice cream into several dessert bowls, sprinkle with pomegranate seeds and raw cacao nibs and serve straight away.

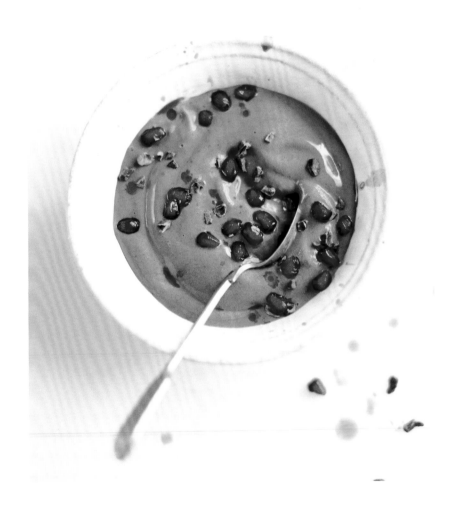

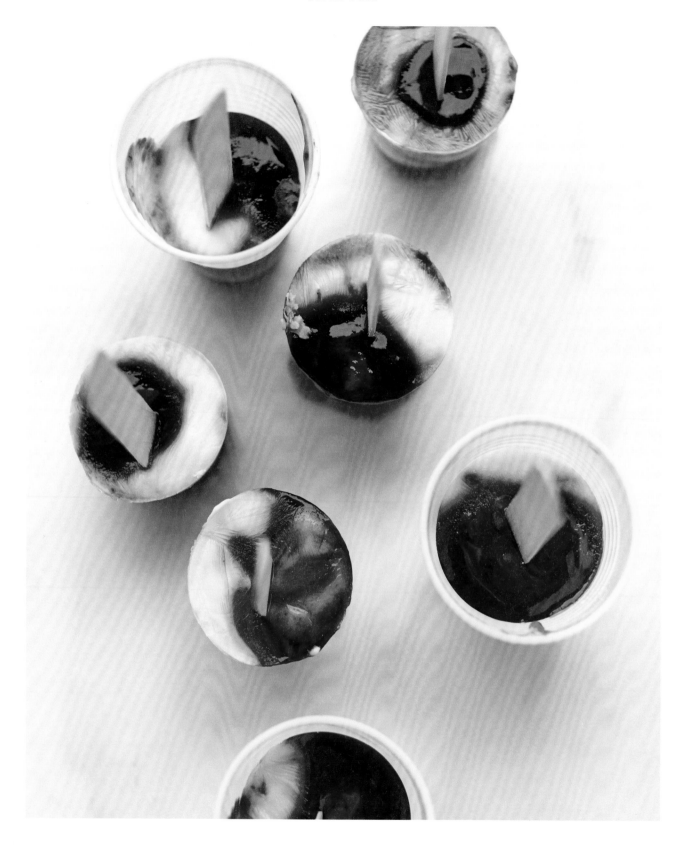

FROZEN YOGHURT
& BLACKBERRY SWIRL POPS

These make for an impressive treat. They are great to make with the kids, perfect for parties or summer barbecues, or just after-school snacks. They are super healthy but super yummy, and kids love them (so do I).

Makes 8
200g blackberries
120g honey, plus an extra 30g
500ml natural yoghurt

8 small disposable plastic cups
8 wooden sticks

Combine the blackberries and the honey in a small saucepan over a gentle heat. Simmer so that the berries cook out and start to become syrupy.

Remove the pan from the heat and blitz the berries with a stick blender, then pass through a sieve and into a clean bowl. Set aside to cool.

Mix the yoghurt and the 30g of honey in a separate large bowl. Gently fold half the cooled berry mix into the yoghurt to create a swirl.

Spoon the mix equally into the plastic cups, pouring a little extra of the purée into the middle of each one. Place the cups into a shallow tray, cover with foil then stick your wooden sticks through the foil into the centre of each cup. The foil will help keep the sticks in place while the pops are freezing. Place the tray in the freezer and freeze for 3–4 hours or until ready to serve. Run the bottom of each cup under hot water to loosen the pop.

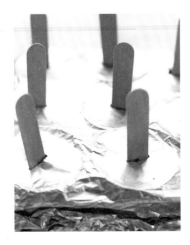

A SUMMERY POMEGRANATE & STRAWBERRY CAKE

Here's a sugar-free cake for celebratory occasions. It's light, fruity, creamy and perfect for a summery afternoon when the strawberries are sweet and fragrant.

Serves 8–10

300g unsalted butter, softened
300g white spelt flour, sifted
4 medium free-range eggs
3 level teaspoons baking powder
2 teaspoons rosewater
300g maple syrup
Grated zest of 1 unwaxed lemon
2–3 tablespoons kefir or milk to loosen the mix

For the filling
250g strawberries
1 pomegranate, halved and seeds removed
Squeeze of lemon juice
400ml double cream
2 tablespoon maple syrup
1 teaspoon rosewater
50g Greek-style natural yoghurt or kefir
6 tablespoons rose petal jam or sugar-free strawberry jam

Preheat the oven to 180°C/gas mark 4. Grease and flour 3 × 20cm loose-bottomed sandwich tins.

In a large mixing bowl, cream the butter until pale and fluffy with an electric hand mixer. Add 2–3 tablespoons of the flour and beat in the eggs, one at a time, and beat until you have a light, fluffy mixture (if it looks as if it's curdling, add another tablespoon of flour). Using a large metal spoon, gently fold in the remaining flour and baking powder until just combined; don't overmix. Add the rosewater, maple syrup and lemon zest, and fold in gently. Add a dash of milk or kefir to loosen if too stiff.

Divide the mixture between the tins, level the top with a palette knife and bake in the oven for 20 minutes or until the centre springs back to the touch. Remove from the oven and cool in the tins for 5–10 minutes before turning out onto a wire rack to cool completely.

Whip the cream until it forms soft peaks, then gently stir through the maple syrup and rosewater. Fold in the yoghurt. Then carefully dot spoonfuls of jam into the cream bowl and give a gentle stir to create a lovely marble effect.

Place one cake layer on a serving plate, gently spoon the cream mixture over and sprinkle with pomegranate seeds. Top with the second cake layer, decorate with marbled cream and pomegranate seeds then repeat a third time with the remaining layer.

Lastly top the cake with your lovely strawberries, sprinkle over any remaining pomegranate seeds. You can also crush a few pomegranate seeds and flick the juice over the cake, this gives a lovely effect.

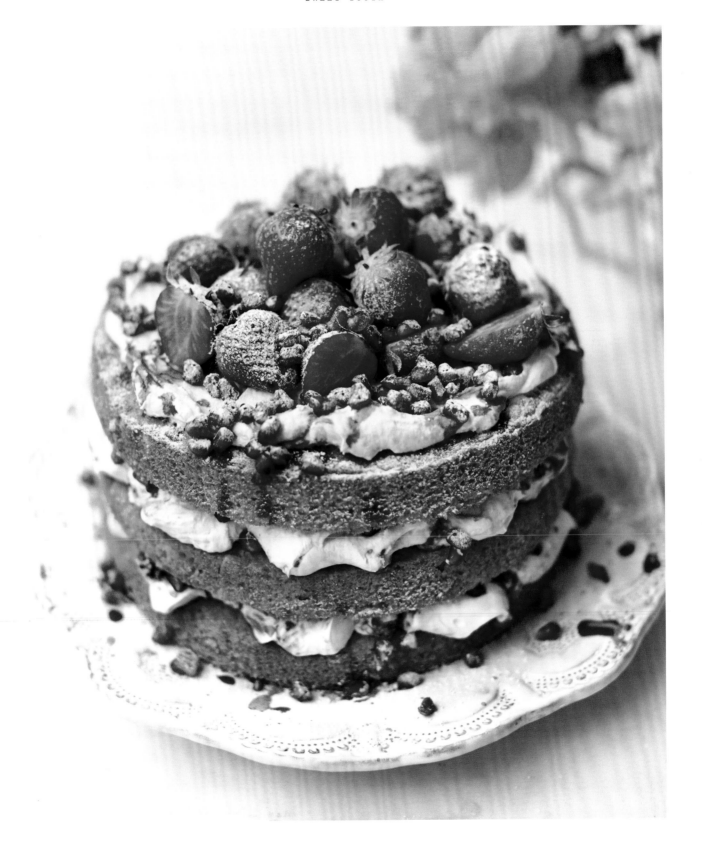

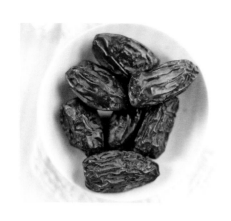

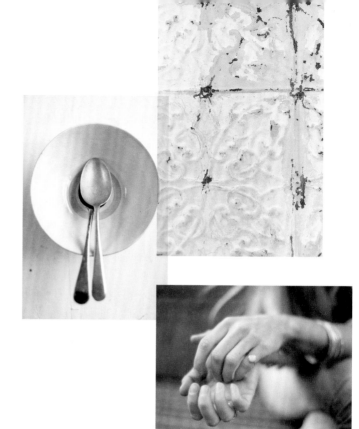

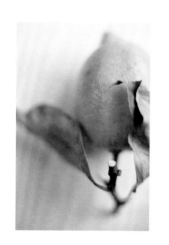

TOOLBOX

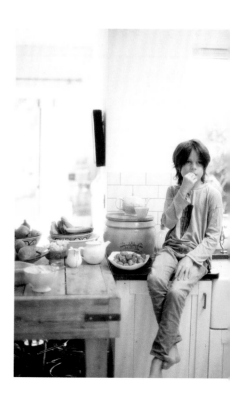

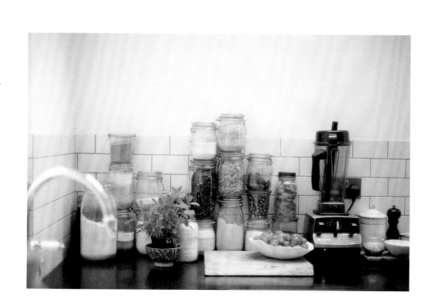

This is my go-to selection of basics, mayos, dressings, dips, sauces etc etc.

You won't believe how easy it is to make these basic things and nothing you buy in the supermarket will compare. I am yet to find a nice pesto sauce from a jar, personally I don't think it exists. However if you prepare your own you can make sure the best and freshest ingredients go into the mix, to end up with something truly health-giving and totally delicious. Mayo has had a bit of a bad reputation, when I think of jar mayo I can understand why; I urge you to try making your own. It's so incredibly good for you, full of healthy fats and proteins. It lasts for a good few days in the fridge and really isn't as tricky as everyone tells you. If you find it splitting simply add a tablespoon of warm water and keep going; it should spring back, no problem.

You can play around with different olive oils for varying degrees of greenness and fruitiness. There are lots of lovely dressings in this chapter, perfect for enhancing any type of salad you have going.

GREMOLATA

I love this stuff: it totally rocks! Anything with gremolata will pop and sing. One small sprinkle elevates the plain to totally genius. I add it to pretty much everything: soups, salads, roasted veg – particularly carrots, parsnips, pumpkins and sweet potatoes – open sandwiches, and use it on meat before or after roasting, fish, chicken. I love it every which way. What's more, it's a great way of using up any parsley that would ordinarily get left in the veg drawer of your fridge and inevitably go yellow and be thrown away, and how many times have we all done that?

Serves enough to sprinkle on a recipe for 4
Bunch of parsley, washed, leaves picked and finely chopped
1 big fat garlic clove or 2 small ones, peeled and finely chopped
2 unwaxed lemons, washed, dried then zested

Simply place all the components into a bowl and toss. That's it, so simple. It keeps well in the fridge for a couple of days but make sure it's sealed with cling film or in an airtight jar.

Variation
My mum grows the most delicious mustard greens. I used to wander through her garden and pick all the baby salad leaves, and mustard greens were one of my faves, deliciously mustardy and peppery. Use them in place of the parsley in the gremolata recipe for a different note.

TARRAGON GREMOLATA

3 tablespoons finely chopped tarragon leaves
Zest of 1 lemon
½ garlic clove, finely chopped

Combine all the ingredients in a small bowl. It will last for only about a day.

HUMMUS

Hummus is a great thing; kids love it, adults love it. I don't know anyone who doesn't. There are some quite good ones you can buy but I much prefer the taste of homemade hummus and that way I know it contains the best quality oils, so no bad fats. Bad fats are one of the worst thing for anyone to eat, especially children. For many reasons, too many to go into here. However, homemade hummus gives you the best of everything, and it tastes far nicer.

Serves 6

400g pre-cooked chickpeas (preferably from a glass jar), drained
4 tablespoons (or more) lemon juice
4 garlic cloves, finely grated
2 teaspoons cumin
Salt to taste
200ml tahini
8 tablespoons water
4 tablespoons extra virgin olive oil, plus a little extra for drizzling
2 teaspoons smoked paprika
2 tablespoons finely chopped curly parsley

Place everything except the paprika and parsley into a blender and blitz until smooth – or put everything in a bowl and use a stick blender, which saves washing up the blender.

Once the mixture is a lovely and creamy, spoon it into a bowl then, using the back of the spoon, carefully smooth it out creating a lovely swirl on the top. Sprinkle over the paprika and parsley, then drizzle a little oil on top.

ROASTED RED PEPPER HUMMUS WITH CHIPOTLE

As left but omit the water and add the flesh of 2 roasted red peppers, skins and seeds removed.
Replace the cumin and paprika and parsley with 1½ teaspoons of chipotle powder.

Finish as above but sprinkle with a little extra chipotle powder.

ROASTED SQUASH & ROSEMARY HUMMUS

As above but omit the water and add 1 cup of roasted butternut squash.
Finish as above but sprinkle with a few rosemary leaves instead of the paprika and parsley.

KALE CRISPS

Kale crisps are perfectly delicious and yet so easy to make. The key is not to have any water on the leaves; if there is moisture they will just wilt in the oven so I tend to wash the leaves the night before and then leave them on the counter on a clean tea towel to dry. You will be surprised how easy these are if you haven't made them before and a lot cheaper than buying them in a shop.

Makes a generous bowlful
1 bunch of kale – 8–10 big leaves
1 tablespoon olive oil
¼ teaspoon sea salt

Optional flavourings
Warming mix
¼ teaspoon turmeric
¼ teaspoon ground cumin
¼ teaspoon ground coriander

Spicy mix
¼ teaspoon chipotle powder
¼ teaspoon oregano

Preheat the oven to 140°C/gas mark 1 and line a baking tray.

Wash the kale leaves and dry them VERY well. Using a paring knife, scissors or simply your hands, strip or cut out and discard the centre stem.

Cut the leaves into 5cm pieces. Put them in a bowl, drizzle with olive oil and sprinkle over the salt. Massage the oil and salt into the leaves until they are well-coated with a thin layer of oil. At this point you can either keep them plain or sprinkle on one of the spice mixes. Spread out the kale on the baking tray and transfer to the oven for 8–12 minutes or until just crisp.

Some of the leaves may crisp faster than others so take out any that are done, then carry on cooking the rest until they are all crisp and lovely. They can be eaten straight away or stored for several days in an airtight tin.

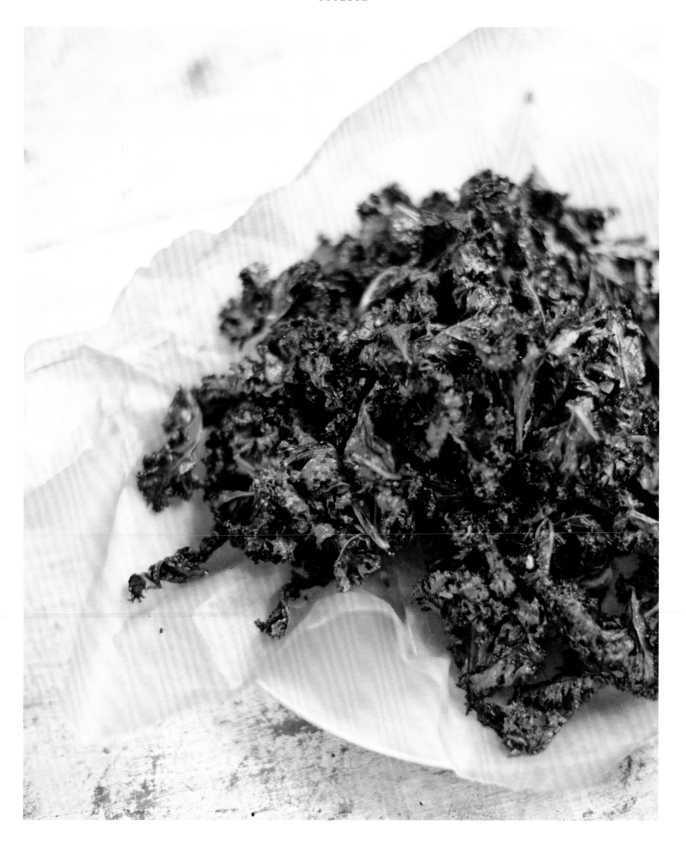

KIMCHI

Kimchi, like sauerkraut, is fermented and very good for you, full of enzymes and probiotics that boost immunity and aid digestion. Try to find Korean red pepper flakes for their slightly sweet, smoky flavour, but otherwise use any red pepper flakes you can find.

Makes 1 large 2.5l jar

1 large Chinese cabbage (also known as Napa cabbage), quartered lengthways, inner cores removed

35g sea salt

Several litres spring water, or mineral water (not tap water, the chlorine will stop the fermentation process)

1 mooli (daikon), peeled and cut into matchsticks

4 spring onions, trimmed and cut into 5cm pieces

For the paste

1 tablespoon grated garlic (about 5 or 6 medium cloves)

1 teaspoon grated ginger

1 teaspoon unrefined sugar

4 tablespoons fish sauce (a good quality one)

1–5 tablespoons Korean red pepper flakes

Cut each cabbage quarter across into 3cm strips and put in a large bowl. Gently massage the salt into the cabbage until it starts to soften a little – 1 or 2 minutes. Add water to cover the cabbage. Put a plate on top and weight it down. Set it aside for 1–2 hours. Pour off the brine into a separate bowl and reserve. Rinse the cabbage under cold water, then let it sit for about 10 minutes in a colander to dry off – pat dry with kitchen towel to remove excess water. Set aside.

Combine the garlic, ginger, sugar and fish sauce in small bowl. Mix in the Korean red pepper flakes, using 1 tablespoon for mild or 5 (or more!) for a fiery taste.

Next take the large bowl used to salt your cabbage, make sure it is clean, and put in all the veg and the paste. Mix with your hands, massaging the seasoning into the veg really well. (Use gloves to protect your hands from chilli or stains or odours.)

Pack the kimchi into a jar, pressing it down well. Pour in enough of the reserved brine to cover the veg completely – it needs to be under the brine. Allow 4cm headspace at the top of the jar. Seal and let it stand at room temperature for 3–5 days, or longer if you're feeling brave! You will see bubbles inside and brine may seep out at the top, so put it in a bowl to catch overflow. Once a day press down the veg to keep them submerged; this releases the gases during fermentation. Taste it daily to check for desired sourness and ripeness.

When the kimchi is to your liking, store the jar in the fridge. You can eat it straight away but it's better if you leave it for a couple of weeks.

MAYONNAISE

Mayo has a bad name after the awful shop-bought varieties have been slathered over even more awful soggy sandwiches. And most of those you buy are terrible for one's health (full of bad fats), in complete contrast to the delicious homemade version (full of good fats). Homemade mayo is actually incredibly good for you, as long as you use the right ingredients: cold-pressed oils and organic free-range eggs – those are good fats with omegas – and in the right ratio. There are SO many delicious ways to use mayo: salads, roast chicken, fish, roast veg, oven roast chips, fish cakes, dressed crab, you name it...

Makes 350ml
2 organic free-range egg yolks
1 teaspoon Dijon mustard
½ tablespoon apple cider vinegar
 or a squeeze of lemon
140ml extra virgin olive oil
145ml cold-pressed sunflower or rapeseed oil
Sea salt and freshly ground pepper

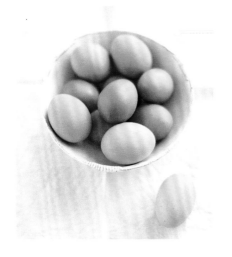

I usually make my mayo by hand, which is easier than you think and saves washing up big pieces of kit. Place a large bowl on a damp cloth on your work surface to hold it secure.

Put the egg yolks in the bowl, add the mustard and vinegar and whisk with a balloon whisk to combine.

Combine the two oils in a separate jug. Pour a very small amount of the oil, only a drop or two, to the yolks and whisk until it's thoroughly combined, then add a tiny bit more oil and whisk again. Keep going in this fashion until quite a bit of oil, which should only take about 3–4 minutes, is incorporated, then start adding more oil at a time. Once I have incorporated the first few drops of oil I add it in a steady trickle with one hand and whisk with the other, stopping every so often to give it a really good whisk before starting the steady trickle again. Once the desired consistency is reached, stop adding the oil (you may not need it all, depending on how you like your mayo). If the mayo starts to split (separate) or you want to thin it a little, add a small amount of warm water.

Now taste it and season as you like it. You can adjust the flavour by adding a little more of the vinegar (or lemon juice) or mustard. It keeps for up to a week in the fridge.

APPLE CIDER VINEGAR

& Raw Honey

This is really good, my go-to dressing for just about any kind of salad or pretty much anything. It keeps very well for a long time.

1 garlic clove, finely grated
1 teaspoon Dijon mustard, heaped
55ml apple cider vinegar
2 tablespoons lemon juice
1–2 tablespoons raw honey – start with one then add more if you like
80ml extra virgin olive oil
Sea salt and freshly ground pepper to taste

Put everything in a jar with a tight-fitting lid or a bowl and either shake or whisk until completely emulsified.

SIMPLEST EVER OLIVE OIL

& Lemon Juice Dressing

This one is for when you just need a little something extra on your veg, but not a full-blown dressing. It's very good and incredibly alkalising.

4 tablespoons extra virgin olive oil
3 tablespoons lemon juice
Sea salt and freshly ground pepper to taste

Simply whisk the oil and lemon in a bowl, season to taste and use immediately.

JAPANESE DRESSING

This one is something a bit different: try it on steamed veg or a carrot and beet salad or Roast Pumpkin, Golden Beets & Squash Salad (see page 59).

70g red onion, finely chopped
3 tablespoons soy sauce
2 tablespoons rice wine vinegar
½ teaspoon raw honey or maple syrup
¼ teaspoon English mustard powder
1 tablespoon grapeseed oil
1 tablespoon sesame oil
Sea salt and freshly ground pepper to taste

Put everything in a jar with a tight-fitting lid, shake really well until completely emulsified then add 2 tablespoons of water. Taste and season accordingly.

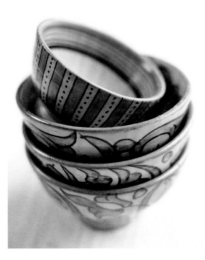

These dressings all make enough for one big salad.

BLACK OLIVE

& Olive Oil Dressing

This is a niçoise dressing for salade niçoise, but as it's quite punchy it goes really well with other bold salads, with potatoes, fish and plenty of other delicious things.

50g black olives, pitted
5 good quality marinated anchovy fillets
1 garlic clove, peeled
Juice of ½ lemon
4 tablespoons olive oil
1 tablespoon apple cider vinegar

Tip the olives, anchovies and garlic into a large mortar and mash with a pestle to make a rough paste. Scrape the mix into a bowl, stir in the lemon juice, olive oil and vinegar and set aside for 10–30 minutes before using so that the flavours can really develop.

ORANGE BLOSSOM

& Maple Syrup Dressing

This dressing is truly amazing on any kind of salad with fruit in it. It really comes alive with the floral notes from the orange blossom water. Be sure to use original Lebanese brands like Cortas which you can find online. Supermarket brands are much more intense so, if using, start by adding ½ teaspoon at a time.

1 tablespoon orange blossom water
2 tablespoons apple cider vinegar
1 tablespoon maple syrup
3 tablespoons olive oil
Juice of ½ lemon
½ garlic clove, finely grated
Sea salt and freshly ground pepper to taste

Combine all the ingredients and whisk in a bowl or shake in a jar with a tight-fitting lid until completely emulsified. Allow to stand for 10 minutes or more before using to allow the flavours to come together.

FRESH ORANGE DRESSING

Another great salad dressing for fruity salads and bitter leaf salads.

Zest and juice of 2 oranges
1 tablespoon apple cider vinegar
1 teaspoon raw honey
Pinch of sea salt and a few twists of freshly ground black pepper
100ml extra virgin olive oil

Put the orange zest and juice in a mixing bowl and stir in the vinegar, honey, salt and pepper. Slowly pour in the oil, a little at a time, whisking continuously to bring it together.

YOGHURT SAUCE

with herb spices

This little gem is amazing with grilled meats, roast chicken, it's wonderful with roast veg and salad. It will make any plate sing.

Enough for 4 as an accompaniment
400g Greek or natural yoghurt
2 fat cloves garlic, peeled and crushed or
  finely grated
1 green chilli, deseeded and finely chopped
6-8 tablespoons dill, stalks removed and
  finely chopped
Sea salt and fresh pepper to taste

Simply put all the ingredients in a bowl and combine. Allow to amalgamate for 15 minutes before using to allow all the flavours really mingle. Taste before serving as often the seasoning will need to be adjusted.

VEG STOCK

Making your own veg stock is really worth the effort. If you're making soups, casseroles or risottos, it's the magic ingredient. It's super easy and good as a vegetable broth, very restorative and healing.

Makes a big bowlful
4 garlic cloves, peeled
2 onions, peeled and cut into quarters
3 carrots, peeled and cut into chunks
2 stalks of celery, each cut into 4 pieces
1 large leek, thoroughly washed and cut into chunks
Handful of flat leaf parsley
4 sprigs of thyme
2 sprigs of fresh tarragon
2 bay leaves
1½ teaspoons salt
1 teaspoon black peppercorns

Place everything into a big pot, cover with 3½-4 litres of water, bring to the boil then reduce the heat and simmer for an hour. Let the stock cool and pour through a strainer, discard all the solids and store the broth in jars in the fridge or freezer.

ROASTED RED PEPPER & ROSEMARY SPREAD

This is so easy to make and totally grain-free. I first came across the idea in The Green Kitchen *by David Frenkiel and Luise Vindahl, and this is my version. I love to keep a jar of it in my fridge at all times, it's perfect with roast veg, or a grilled piece of fish, or as a spread on rye toast with avocado and salad or even as dip with seasonal crudités. The seeds add lots of good oils and in particular the pumpkin seeds have lots of zinc which is great for balancing the hormones and clearing the skin.*

Makes 1 x 500g jar
3 red bell peppers, halved and deseeded
Olive oil
2 sprigs of rosemary leaves picked
50g sunflower seeds
50g pumpkin seeds
Pinch of smoked paprika
Juice of ½ lemon
A hearty pinch of sea salt
Freshly ground black pepper

Preheat your oven to 200°C/gas mark 6.

Place the prepared peppers onto a flat roasting tray and drizzle with olive oil. Sprinkle over the rosemary and toss. Roast for about 40 minutes or until slightly charred at the edges and the skin is easy to peel off. Set aside to cool.

Next lightly toast the seeds in a dry frying pan, until they start to release their delicious nutty aroma and they are starting to pop. Transfer them to a bowl.

When the peppers are cool enough to handle, peel off the skins. Place them into a bowl along with the rest of the ingredients and blitz until smooth. Taste and adjust the seasoning if necessary. Scrape your mix into a glass jar and keep in the fridge for up to 2 weeks, if it lasts that long!! Mine never does.

DUKKAH

This Egyptian spice blend is glorious sprinkled onto an omelette or scrambled eggs, or on avocado on toast. It's goes well on roast chicken, or with fish. Serve a small bowlful alongside one with good quality olive oil in it and a pile of fresh, hot whole grain pitta breads. It keeps for ages on the shelf in an air tight jar but it's so good it won't be around for long.

Makes 1 medium jarful
130g hazelnuts
40g coriander seeds
6 teaspoons sesame seeds
4 tablespoons cumin seeds
2 tablespoons balck peppercorns
2 teaspoons fennel seeds
2 teaspoons dried mint leaves
2 teaspoons flaky sea salt

Heat a heavy-bottomed pan over a high heat, add the hazelnuts and dry roast until slightly browned and fragrant, being careful not to let them burn, which they can do easily. Remove from the heat and cool completely.

Repeat the procedure with each of the seeds and peppercorns, subsequently allowing each to cool completely.

Place the nuts, seeds, mint and salt into a mortar or small spice blender and bound or blitz until the mix is a course consistency. Do NOT allow the mix to become a paste; you want a lovely crumbly spice mix. Delicious.

MY MUM'S PLUM SAUCE

This is the sauce I grew up on. I LOVE it!! If I had to choose 5 favourite tastes from my childhood this would be one of them. We had it on everything from fish and chips through to shepherd's pie, or with our delicious home made sausages. My mum always had the shelves stocked with this sauce. It's like a plum version of a tomato sauce, rather than the thick sweet chinese plum sauce. Use it as you would ketchup. Half the recipe is good the first time until you're addicted, like me!

Makes enough to last you 6 months
3.5kg dark red tart plums, halved and pitted
1.5kg rapadura (evaporated cane juice)
2 teaspoons sea salt
1 teaspoon allspice berries
1 teaspoon whole cloves
115g grated ginger
2l apple cider vinegar

Place everything into a large, heavy-bottomed pot, bring to the boil and simmer for 2 hours. Set aside to cool completely. When it's cooled to room temperature, pour into sterilised bottles with sealing lids or tops. This sauce will keep well for months if sealed properly.

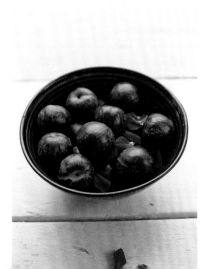

PESTO

a few ways

Pesto is great as a dip, as sauce for roast veg, as a dressing or on sandwiches, even on rye toast with a delicious soft cheese.....it's full of good fats to feed the brain and herbs which aid digestion and give many micro nutrients that feed the body on a deep level.

CLASSIC PESTO

Makes enough for 3–4
½ clove of garlic, chopped
3 handfuls of freshly washed basil leaves, picked and chopped
1 handful of pinenuts, lightly toasted
1 hearty handful of parmesan (or a mature pecorino), finely grated
150ml extra virgin olive oil
Small squeeze of lemon juice
Sea salt and freshly ground pepper

Add the garlic, basil, pine nuts, parmesan and olive oil into a food processor and blitz it to a rough sauce; I don't like it too smooth. You may add a little extra oil if you like it more runny. Add a squeeze of lemon, just a small one and season to taste.

WALNUT PESTO WITH BASIL OR KALE

Makes enough for 3–4
175g walnut halves or pieces
1 garlic clove
Handful of fresh basil (or kale)
100g parmesan, freshly grated
100ml extra-virgin olive oil
Sea salt and pepper

Place everything into a blender and blitz until you have a rough sauce. Adjust the balance with a little extra cheese or oil. Season to taste.

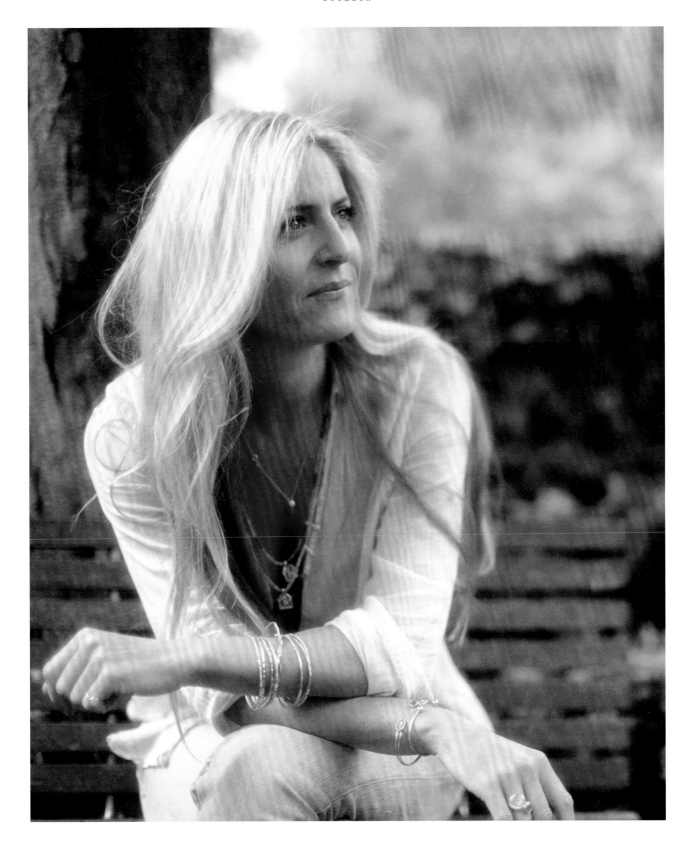

SOFT, FRESHLY WHIPPED CREAM

This is perfect for topping fruit pies and puddings, fruit salad with a sprinkle of my rosewater granola, heaven or even as a topping for my coconut and banana pancakes with a sugar-free jam. You can use this cream in so many ways.

500ml fresh cream
3 tablespoons natural yoghurt or kefir
2 tablespoons raw honey or raw date syrup (see page 119)

Whip the cream to ribbon consistency, gently fold in the yoghurt or kefir and honey or syrup with a spatula. If you like your cream a little stiffer, just beat a little more until you achieve the desired thickness but don't overwhip.

RICH MASCARPONE CREAM

Use this as you would the softly whipped cow's cream. It's great for people who are avoiding dairy, its vegan friendly and it tastes totally indulgent! I love eating this with my Som Tum Pollami fruit salad (see page 47).

500g mascarpone or soured cream
3 free-range egg yolks
120g maple syrup or raw honey or raw date syrup (see page 119)

Beat the mascarpone lightly in a bowl. Beat the egg yolks in a separate bowl and slowly add the maple syrup. Fold in the mascarpone. Chill in the fridge.

LIGHT, COCONUT CREAM

with Vanilla

This is good with baked fruits, hot from the oven it will melt into the hot fruit and create a lovely melty sauce, total heaven! It's also good on cakes as an icing.

1 x 400ml tin full-fat coconut cream
1 teaspoon raw honey or raw date syrup (see page 119), or to taste
Seeds from ¼ vanilla pod

Place the tin of coconut milk upside down in the fridge for several hours or overnight. Turn the tin the right way up, open and pour off the thin coconut water into a bowl or small jar and set aside for another use.

Spoon out the thick cream in the bottom of the tin into a medium bowl, add the honey and vanilla seeds then whip with a whisk or electric beaters for about 3–5 minutes until light and fluffy like whipped cream. If it's too thick, you can add 1–2 teaspoons of the reserved coconut water to make it lighter and smoother. Taste and add more honey if you like.

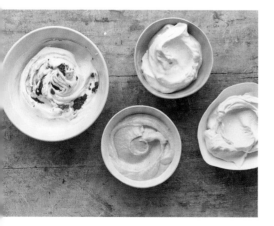

THICK, LOVELY CASHEW CREAM

This cream is really velvety and nutty and creamy, totally luscious. It's a great non dairy alternative but even if you are having dairy I still choose this sometimes; it's a treat unto itself. It's beautiful with baked fruits and on top of cakes.

160g cashew nuts, soaked for at least 4 hours or overnight
1–2 tablespoons raw honey or raw date syrup or to taste
Seeds from ¼ vanilla pod
120ml water
Pinch of sea salt

Put the cashew nuts, with 1 tablespoon of the honey, the vanilla seeds and salt into a high speed blender. Add two-thirds of the water and blitz, scraping down the sides if necessary, until it's lovely and velvety and smooth. If it's too thick, add more water to thin it out to desired consistency. Taste and add more honey if you like.

Variation
For a fruit version of any of these creams, use a fork to mash a few perfectly ripe in-season berries – raspberries, blackberries, boysenberries, loganberries, blackcurrants and redcurrants all work well, strawberries less so; they're too watery) – then marble them through the cream before serving.

RAW DATE SYRUP

Medjool dates have a deep, sweet flavour that makes them a perfect alternative to processed sugar when you need a natural sweetener.

10 medjool dates, pitted (or 20 normal dates, pitted)
420 ml luke warm water
1 teaspoon fresh lemon juice

Start by soaking the dates in the water overnight, covered. Then place them in a blender, together with the soaking water and lemon juice and blitz until completely smooth. Transfer to a jar with a lid and store in the fridge; it keeps for up to 3 weeks.

If you don't like the pips, mash the fruit with a fork then push the mix through a sieve, discard the pips and marble the pulp and liquid through the cream.

NUT MILK

This is a great alternative to dairy milk. It's easy to make and so delicious.

1 cup almonds
2 cup fresh water (filtered or spring water is best)

Start by soaking you nuts overnight in a bowl. The nuts should be covered with water by at least an inch. The next day, drain the nits and place them in a blender. Blitz them for 2 minutes.

Take a cheese cloth or nut milk bag and place it over a bowl. Pour in the blitzed nut milk mixture and then, with clean hands, squeeze the liquid through the cloth into the bowl, extracting as much mulk as possible. You should have about 2 cups of milk. You now have ground almonds left in the cloth, which you can use for baking.

Pour your nut milk into a jar with a lid and store in the fridge to keep it cool until you are ready to use it. It will last in the fridge for a couple of days, but you will need to give it a good shake before using.

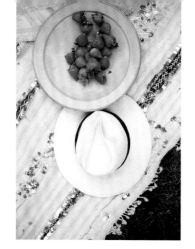
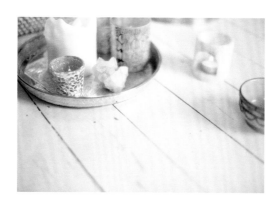
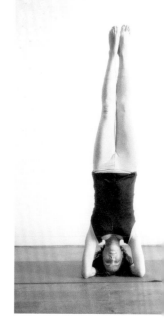
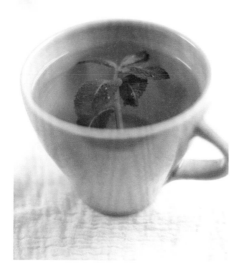
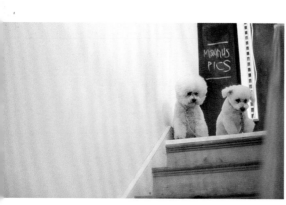
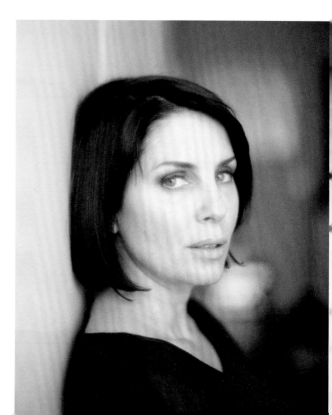

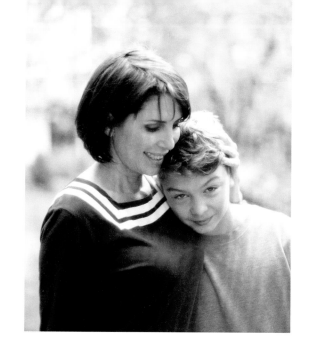

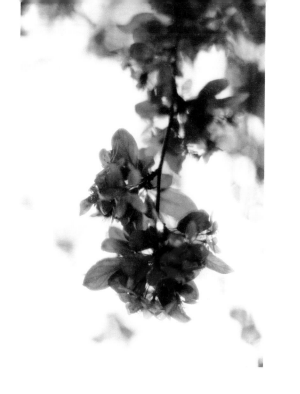

SUPER-WOMAN

Sadie

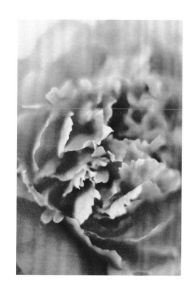

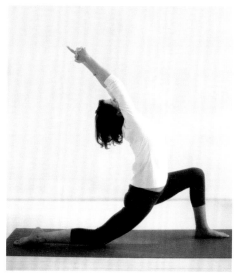

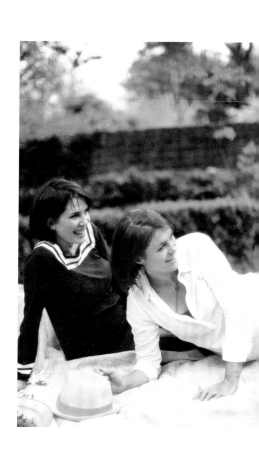

From my earliest memories, diet and exercise have been very important to me. Taking care of my body has been a very natural process that has come easily, so in some ways I have been lucky. I was a natural vegetarian, from the start; as a child I chose not to eat meat as I intensely disliked the taste of both meat and fish. My childhood was spent exercising, dancing and doing gymnastics, always pushing myself to the limit. All of this physical activity gave me a great start and a solid foundation for living healthily.

I've always strived to do my best, to challenge myself and to try my utmost to be positive and content. Of course, as I have found out, getting a certain amount of balance in life isn't always easy and it is quite possible to lose your way and become disillusioned and unmotivated. Life doesn't always bring contentment, happiness and peace of mind. For every one of us it's a journey: we can be up or down, we can be happy or sad, positive or negative. So many people suffer from anxiety, depression and/or feelings of worthlessness at some point in life and I too have experienced all of these, which led me to explore many avenues to find some contentment.

I wanted to use my part of the book to outline how I conquered my demons. My aim is to share what I have learnt from my experience in an approachable and unintimidating way…

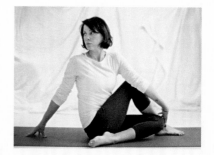

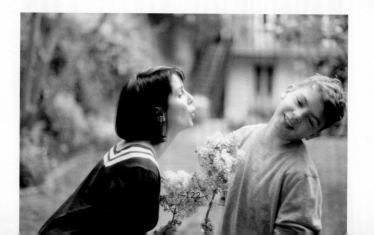

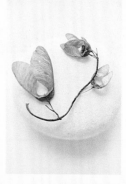

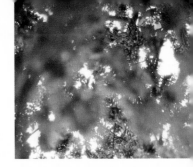

I wanted to use my part of the book to outline how I conquered my demons. My aim is to share what I have learnt from my experience in an approachable and unintimidating way, giving you the same insights I have gained from those who have taught and helped me over the years.

To live in the moment is vital. I used to spend so much of my life rushing around, never present, never listening, always on the phone or distracted. Listening is a very important skill and something I have always had to work on. Even normal human functions were a strain – eating, sleeping and just living were all tasks that I found very difficult. How, I wondered, could I change? I ate right, I exercised and, yet, it still felt like there was something wrong with me. I saw healers, homeopaths, acupuncturists, gurus, and meditation experts. The number of specialists I visited was endless – a full-time job really! But each time I saw someone I took a little bit of their thinking away with me and eventually I put together my own little plan for mind, body and soul that I now try to practise every day. It's a plan that fits into my normal routine because I am a working mum with a lot on, not someone living on a mountain or taking time out on a yoga retreat. Of course, I am far from perfect and sometimes my plan falls apart into a million pieces. But each time this happens it is becoming easier to pick myself up, dust myself down and start again.

When you experience peace of mind and contentment, it is the most wonderful feeling in the world, as if warm treacle is running through your veins. There is a certain detachment, a sitting back and letting go. You feel alert, yet slightly fuzzy like on one of those perfect summer days when you feel totally blissed out and loved. You can sit and listen to people and take it all in, without your mind churning through pointless thoughts.

The plan I have developed uses a combination of yoga, meditation, mindfulness and good eating. It is a daily practice of positivity, assertiveness and surrender that nurtures the mind, body and soul and it begins with the way you breathe.

Love,
Sadie x

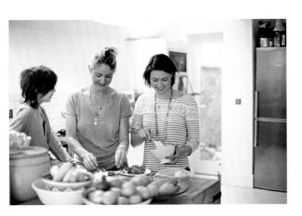

BREATH

Breath is everything! It gives us energy, life, and, if we are breathing properly, contentment and calmness. We can go for some time without water, food and sleep but breath is essential. How we breathe can rapidly rejuvenate us and connect us to our life-force. In yoga practice 'breath' is called 'pranyama', 'prana' meaning life force and 'yama' extension. So the translation of pranyama is 'extension of life-force'. It can help engage our body and mind in times of need.

As a young child I suffered from a condition called bronchiectasis, which meant I had breathing difficulties. I was subjected to panic attacks and anxiety because I was not truly connected to my breath. Once I started to learn how important it was to breathe properly I became calmer and more in control and at peace with myself. Over the years I have learnt many breathing techniques from lots of people, from voice coaches, singing teachers and finally from some of the best yoga teachers I could find, which was when I really began to understand breath and the power of it. When you control the inhalation and exhalation of breath it purifies and cleans your body. Immediately breathing can calm your mind and at the same time give you energy.

When I wake up in the morning I slowly open my eyes. I try to focus on the moment, not on the hectic day I may have ahead of me. I start by engaging with pranyama and a light meditation along with some of my favourite mantras, saying something such as 'I am content in the now' or 'I love and support myself.' This means I start my day in a serene, calm and connected way and, hopefully, my whole day will be focused and enjoyable. I really notice a difference; I have clarity of thought and I am calm. If I don't do this it can be a whole other story, which sees me rushing around like a headless chicken worrying about the kids and my busy schedule.

So, in a very simple way, I will explain how I use my breath in some exercises.

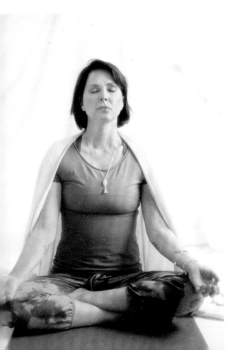
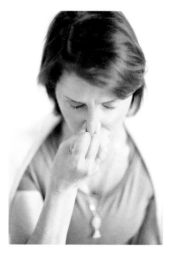

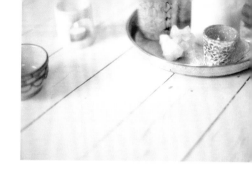

TYPES *of* BREATH

Ujjayi (u-jai-yee)

Ujjayi, meaning hissing, is one of my favourite types of breath. It is also called the sounding breath due to the huffing sound you make as you exhale. When I breathe in this way it makes me feel energised, focused and improves my concentration in the physical practice. Becoming absorbed in Ujjayi allows you to remain in a yoga pose for longer periods of time. It also enhances more of a flow to the practice. Ujjayi breathing also helps to cure respiratory conditions such as asthma and bronchitis.

Sit up straight, close your eyes and breath naturally.

When you are ready to begin, take a deep breath in through your nose. Let the breath flow through your body. As you exhale, constrict your throat slightly so that there is a tension there, and then release the breath from the tension in your throat to create a *haaa* sound. Imagine you are cleaning a pair of glasses and huff on the lense, as it is a similar action and sound.

Inhale again and, as you did before, let the tension in your throat create the same *haaa* sound as you exhale. Once you have got the hang of this, close your mouth and breathe through your nostrils. You should now start to sound like Darth Vader!

Once you have mastered this on the exhale, use the tension in your

throat to create the same breath and sound on the inhale too. (You truly will sound like Darth Vader now!)

Breath of Fire

Breath of Fire is a breathing technique that is used to boost your energy as it oxygenates and detoxifies the blood. It also aids brain function and concentration. It is great for calming the nervous system and for giving a sense of well-being, although some recommend not to practise it if you are pregnant or menstruating. The best time to perform breath of fire is in the morning, or a few hours after eating when your food has digested.

To begin, take some normal deep breaths, then start to inhale and exhale rapidly through your nose, keeping the length of the inhale and exhale equal. You will notice your stomach contract with some force.

Another way to start is by sticking your tongue out and panting like a dog. Then close your mouth and continue breath and rhythm, rapidly inhaling and exhaling through your nose. This sets up a good rhythm to stick with. Use your abdomen to inhale and exhale, pulling it in tightly and then pumping out the air just like using a set of bellows.

For best results, try to practise Breath of Fire for 1 to 4 minutes each day if possible.

Alternate Nostril Breathing

Daily alternate nostril breathing is incredibly beneficial to your well-being. Ancient Yogis, who practised yoga thousands of years ago, believed that many diseases were connected to irregular nasal breathing. As your nose is directly linked to your brain, alternate nasal breathing allows both sides of the brain to function optimally, which in turn calms the mind. Its other benefits include improving sleep, boosting the pineal gland, balancing hormones and calming the nervous system.

Simply inhale through the left nostril, while closing the right with your thumb. Hold the breath, covering both nostrils. Release your right nostril and exhale.

Now inhale through your right nostril, again hold the breath covering both nostrils and then exhale through your left nostril.

This counts as one round: you can either do it slowly in your own time or inhale for the count of 4, hold for 10 and exhale for 8. Try to do 6–10 rounds every day for 21 days and notice the difference.

BREATHING EXERCISES

Breathing to Relax

During times of stress it is common for us to tighten our chest, grip our shoulders and shorten our exhalations, even to the point of not exhaling at all so that we are holding our breath.

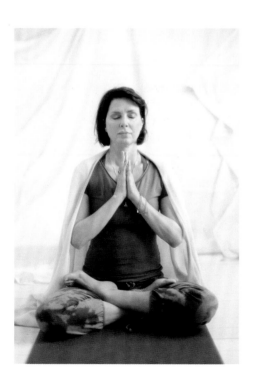

How to do breathing to relax

To enhance relaxed breathing, you need to consciously relax your chest, shoulders, neck, jaw and tongue. Then imagine the breath easily flowing and filling the deepest parts of your lungs. Bring awareness to your breath. The speed and depth will alternate – just observe this without trying to change a thing. Simply focusing on your breath can create a calm and serene state of being. To achieve this, move your belly with each breath. When you inhale, the diaphragm descends towards your abdomen, which pushes the abdominal muscles and gently swells your belly. As you exhale, the diaphragm releases back towards the heart, enabling the belly to release towards the spine.

For a quick and effective way to relax through a stressful situation, breathe in through your nose, keeping your mouth closed and tongue relaxed, holding for the count of 4, then when you have finished inhaling, hold for the count of 2 and then slowly exhale to the count of 6.

Viparita Karani

Another good exercise for calming is to lie with your bottom against a wall and your legs up the wall at a right angle. To get in this position you will need to sit on the floor facing the wall and manoeuvre your legs up the wall and wriggle yourself so that your bum touches the wall. Remain in this position for 15 minutes doing nothing, just sitting with yourself and breathing. This will make you feel centred and filled with contentment.

WE ALL NEED TO BREATHE, OF COURSE IF WE DIDN'T WE WOULD DIE! BECOMING AWARE OF HOW BREATHING CHANGES UNDER DIFFERENT CIRCUMSTANCES AND TEACHING YOURSELF TO BREATHE PROPERLY ARE SOME OF THE MOST SIMPLE, YET BENEFICIAL THINGS YOU CAN DO FOR YOURSELF. THE AIM OF THESE EXERCISES IS TO KEEP YOU RELAXED AND CALM THROUGH ALL THE UPS AND DOWNS OF LIFE.

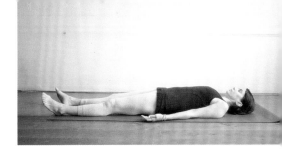

Breathing to Sleep

This is a very quick and thorough way of inducing sleep. You start with your relaxation breath, and then expand your breath so that you feel as if you are breathing your awareness into your entire body. As you breathe in, allow the breath to reach every part of your body – beginning with your feet.

How to do breathing to sleep

Take your breath and awareness to your toes and feet and silently say to yourself 'I relax my toes and feet, my toes and feet are relaxed and happy.' Then switch your focus up to your calves and give them your breath and attention. Slowly move your breath and awareness up through your whole body, including all your inner organs, until you are breathing into your head, brain, and the top of your scalp.

Hopefully by this point you will be asleep but if for any reason you're not then breathe into your head and as you exhale imagine all your worries and thoughts releasing through the top of your head.

Breathing to Energise

I recommend you repeat this exercise three times a day as a general strengthener and to sustain energy and good health.

How to do breathing to energise

Using deep, hearty breaths here, breathing through the nose again, mouth closed and with your tongue relaxed: breathe in for the count of 2, hold for the count of 4, and breathe out for 2 counts. Repeat this sequence of breaths 10 times.

Breathing to Focus the Mind

Another exercise I find very helpful if I am feeling anxious is to get into the yoga position known as Downward Facing Dog. To me this exercise is extremely valuable. I use it if I need to be energised, if I'm angry, confused, in fact in any emotional state. It can be incredibly beneficial.

Get onto your hand and knees, setting your knees directly below your hips and your hands slightly forward of your shoulders. Make sure your palms are spread, your fingers parallel or slightly turned out and your toes are turned under.

Now exhale and lift your knees away from the floor, ensuring your tailbone is lengthened away from the back of your pelvis. Do ten deep breaths, in through your nose, out through your nose, making that Darth Vader sound I described earlier as if you are brushing the back of your throat with your breath.

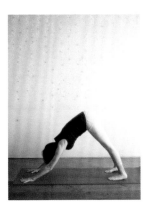

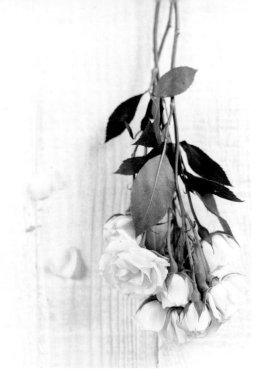

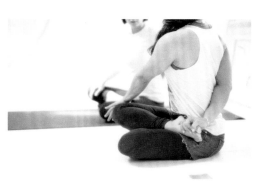

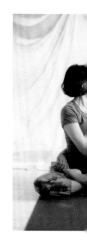

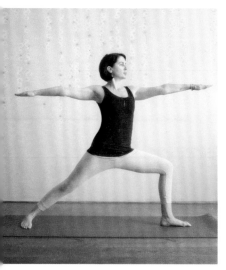

YOGA

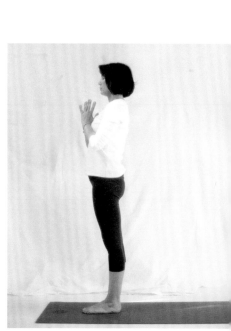

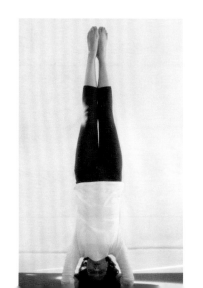

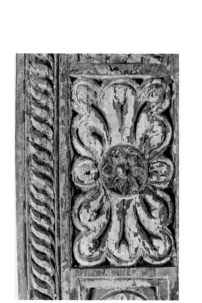

I was first introduced to yoga by my mother when I was 15 as she thought it would help with the breathing difficulties I had always had as a child. I took some classes and enjoyed them immensely but it took me a long time to truly get it and to fully understand what yoga does and what its benefits are. In my mid-teens I was just too restless and unable to concentrate. Many years later after numerous classes, courses and instructions from some of the best teachers in the world, I feel I can finally incorporate yoga into my daily life without it being a chore and now it brings me only joy and a sense of calm.

Yoga has been practised for at least 2,500 years when an Indian author named Patanjali wrote the yoga sutras, which constituted the first yoga text known to be written. He defined yoga as *chitta-vrtta-nirohdah*, which means the cessation of the turning of the mind. This is exactly what it means to me: a calming of the mind, so that the washing machine head I can sometimes have slows down and stops. The postures physically stretch and tone your body, of course, keeping it young and supple, but the higher aim is to connect with the universe so your mind, body and soul are all at one. The inner stillness is fantastic.

Yoga does many things for you. It stimulates your glands and cleanses your vital organs. It creates a flexible and strong body, improves respiration, energy, and vitality, helps to maintain a balanced metabolism, promotes cardio and circulatory health, relieves pain, helps you look and feel younger and improves your athletic performance.

TYPES *of* YOGA

There are many different schools of yoga and I have tried nearly all of them. It is a personal choice which you prefer; the end results and benefits are more or less the same.

01 Ashtanga (or Astanga)
Ashtanga is the name given to the system of yoga taught by Sri K. Pattabhi Jois. Physically it is demanding as it involves synchronising breathing with a progressive and continuous series of postures. This process produces intense internal heat and a profuse, purifying sweat that detoxifies muscles and organs. The result is improved circulation, flexibility, stamina and a calm mind. I find Ashtanga can be highly addictive as you zone out completely when practising the repetitive routine.

02 Dharma Mittra
Dharma Mittra is a very physical sequence that involves a lot of balancing, twisting, stretching and back bends. It feels quite athletic or contemporary dance based. These sequences are a little different to other types of yoga and more intense; I recommend you try this if you are advanced at practising yoga.

03 Hatha
This is the first type of yoga I tried. I always feel that Hatha is the gentlest form of yoga, making it a good one to start with. It uses postures (asanas) and stretches in combination with the breath to develop flexibility and relaxation. There are many styles of Hatha yoga. It brings balance, strength and calmness.

01

02

03

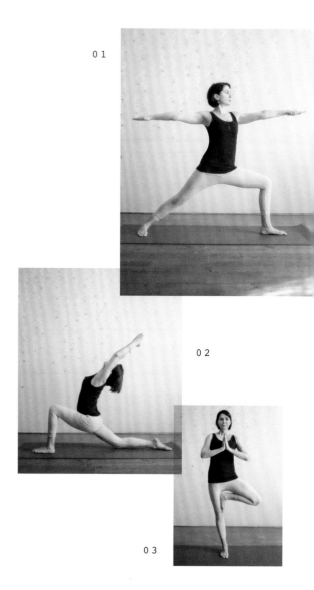

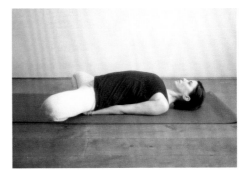

04

04 Iyengar

This type of yoga is taught by trying to get every pose exactly correct and with complete alignment. Iyengar teachers believe that one day their students will be able to attain perfect poses through constant practice and that, once they have created the balance in the body, it will be reflected in the mind. Iyengar yoga uses a lot of props – blocks, bolsters, chairs, pillows, and straps.

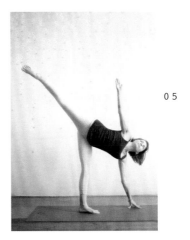

05

05 Jivamukti

Jivamukti is a vinyasa-style, meaning alignment of yoga and breath. Practice and classes are physically quite intense. Each class has a theme, which is explored through yoga scripture, chanting, meditation, asana (yoga postures) pranyama and music. Jivamukti appeals to those who want a good workout and also something to stretch their minds because it includes chanting and philosophising. Jivamukti classes can be quite diverse in style and more fun than lots of other classes, and almost feel like you're in a rave!

06 Kundalini

The word *kundalini* refers to the coiled energy of the Root chakra, which surrounds the base of the spine. The principle behind Kundalini yoga is that by freeing up this area, we can unleash the unlimited potential that lies within that energy centre. Kundalini can be quite intense and challenging and is a more spiritual style of yoga. It focuses on specific breathing techniques that intensify the effects of the poses with the purpose of freeing energy in the lower body and allowing it to move upwards.

06

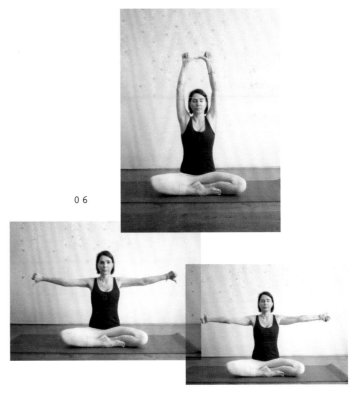

your

DAILY PRACTICE

I try to practise yoga every day for 20–30 minutes, and then maybe one 90-minute lesson a week. By doing just 20 minutes a day you get the benefit without having to squeeze too much time into your diary.

This is not a specialist yoga book, but I wanted to include the exercises I couldn't do without that help with moods and emotions. Try to find a local yoga class where you can practise regularly. If you can't, try a recommended yoga book or DVD and practise at home.

Surya Namaskara (Sun Salutation)
There are many different types of sun salutation. This is my favourite because it feels dynamic and complete. The continuous flowing builds heat in the body whilst raising your heart rate. Each pose coordinates with your breath, you inhale to extend and exhale to bend.

01 Stand in Tadasana (see page 137). Make sure your feet are grounded and the weight is distributed evenly. Bring your hands into prayer position at your heart's center and gently close your eyes and start ujjayi breath.

02 Inhale through your nose and stretch your arms out to the side and overhead into Urdhva Hastasana (Upward Salute). Look upwards towards the ceiling.

03 As you exhale, fold into Uttanasana (standing forward bend). Make sure your spine is straight (you can bend your knees if you need to). Keep your legs engaged and draw your kneecaps towards you.

04 Inhale and lengthen your spine forwards into Ardha Uttanasana (Half Standing Forward Bend). Lift your gaze ahead, extend and lengthen the spine. Either place the fingertips on the floor or onto your shins.

05 As you exhale, either step or lightly jump back into plank pose. Your hands should be shoulder distance apart and your feet hip distance. Inhale and lengthen.

06 Exhale and lower into Chaturanga Dandasana (Four-limbed staff pose). Either keep your legs straight and push back into your heels or bring your knees to the floor.

07 Inhale and bring your chest forward into Urdhya Mukha Svanasana (Upward-facing dog). Make sure you pull your shoulders back and down and lengthen your collarbones, gaze upwards and lengthen neck.

08 As you exhale, roll over the toes and come into Adho Mukha Svanasana (Downward-facing dog pose). Ground through your hands and feet and push your heels towards the floor. Lengthen your spine and stay here for five breaths. Enjoy this moment.

09 Exhale, bend your knees and look between your hands. As you inhale, either step or lightly hop your feet between your hands, returning to Ardha Uttanasana.

10 Exhale back to Uttanasana.

11 As you inhale, reach your arms out wide to your sides and come to stand, ensuring your back is lengthening. Draw your arms overhead to Urdhva Hastasana and gently bring them back into prayer position at your heart's centre. You can either stay here for a few breaths or go straight into the next sun salutation.

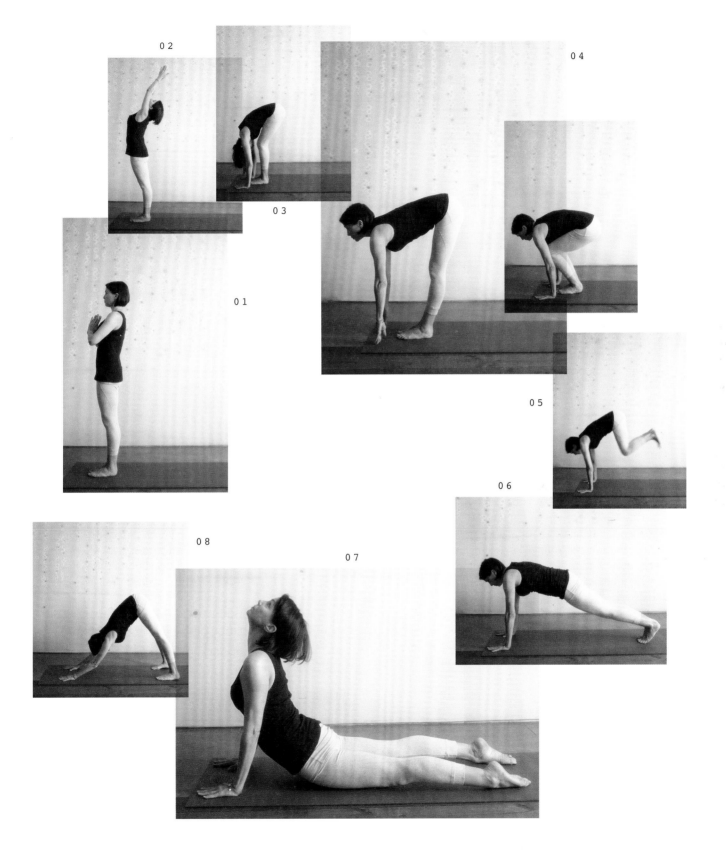

yoga for

DEPRESSION

Yoga works for depression and sadness because it promotes deep relaxation. This is achieved by the controlled breathing during the physical poses (asanas). The heart rate is reduced, blood pressure is lowered and respiration eases. These effects in turn reduce anxiety, depression and anger.

01 Uttanasana (Forward fold)
B.K.S. Iyengar, the founder of Iyengar yoga, writes about Uttanasana in his book Light on Yoga: *'Any depression felt in the mind is removed if one holds the pose for two minutes or more.' You will really benefit from using this standing pose to lift your mood.*

Stand up straight in Tadasana (see page 137). Exhale and bend forward from the hip joints and not the waist. Lengthen your torso, so you can move more freely into the position. With your knees straight or slightly bent, bring your palms or finger tips beside or in front of your feet with your palms to the back of your ankles. Now with your inhalations and exhalations, lift and lengthen your torso and release a little bit more into the forward bend. Here try resting for 2 minutes, then, when you want to come out of this pose, bring your hands back onto your hips. Lengthen your torso and come up in an inhalation to your standing position.

02 Janu Sirsasana (Head-to-knee forward bend)
This yoga position is seated. It is a gentle fold that calms the mind. It also stretches the hamstrings and groin, and stimulates the liver and kidneys.

In a seated position make sure your buttocks are lifted (you can use a folded blanket for this). Position your legs straight in front of you. Inhale and bend your right knee, placing your heel towards the perineum. Rest the sole of your right heel against your left thigh with your right knee close to the floor. From here, hinge forward with your hips, lengthening your spine, with your hands on either side of your right foot. Make sure you don't round your back. Keep looking towards your toes and, by hinging at your waist, your head will be close to your right knee. Breathe deeply in this position for 1–3 minutes then repeat the pose on the opposite side.

03 Bhujangasana (Cobra)

This asana is a backbend that can be done in stages. It expands the chest and gives elasticity to the lungs. The pose resembles the cobra with its hood raised.

Lie on your stomach with your toes flat on the floor and your forehead resting on the ground. Keep your legs close together and your feet and heels lightly touching each other. Place your palms underneath your shoulders, keeping your elbows parallel and close to your torso. Inhale and lift your head, chest and abdomen while keeping your navel on the floor. Keep breathing with awareness, and try to straighten your arms by arching your back as much as possible. Tilt your head and look up. Make sure your shoulders are away from your ears. When you are ready to come out of the pose, gently lower your abdomen, chest and head back to the ground.

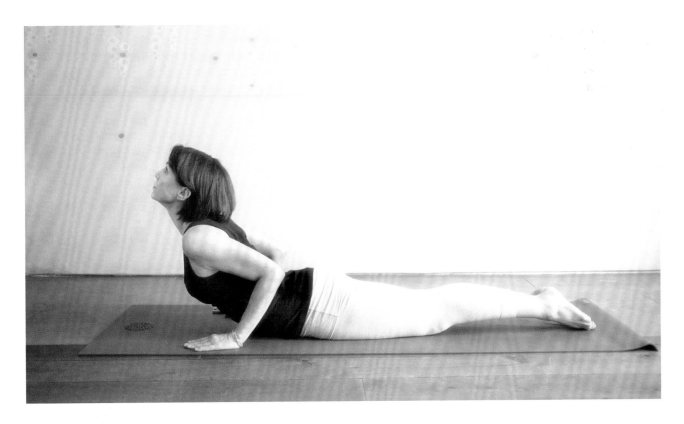

Sirsasana (Headstand)

Performing a headstand would be a valuable addition to your daily practice. Not only does it have physical benefits, the emotional ones are tremendous. Inverting yourself reverses the action of gravity on your body; it changes any negative emotions and leaves you feeling a lot better about things.

The headstand stimulates the pituitary glands to produce endorphins, which act to block pain and increase self-esteem. Beginners can start by doing a headstand against a wall.

Use a mat to pad your head and forearms. Kneel on the floor. Interlock your fingers together and place your forearms on the floor, elbows at shoulder width. Roll your upper arms slightly outwards, pressing your inner wrists into the floor. Place the crown of your head on the floor.

While inhaling, lift your knees off the floor, walking your feet closer to your elbows, heels elevated. Actively lift through the top of your thighs to form an inverted V. Firm your shoulder blades against your back and lift them towards your tailbone so the front torso stays as long as possible (see photo 01). This should help prevent the weight of your shoulders collapsing onto your neck and head.

Gently lift your legs up into the air, aligning your body into a straight line.

Try to hold the pose for 20 breaths, or practise staying up for a longer period each time and work towards that.

When you are ready to come down, slowly lower your legs and stay in Child's Pose (see photo 02).

0 1

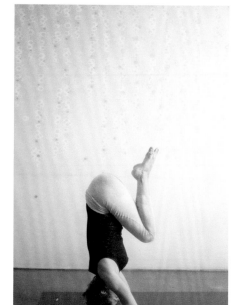

0 2

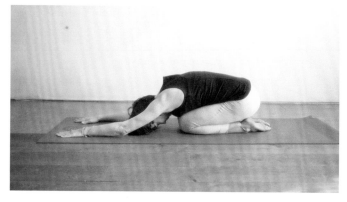

yoga for

CALMING

Tadasana (Mountain pose)

If you feel upset or overwrought, you need a pose that helps you stay focused and grounded. An awareness of your feet being connected to the floor is very calming.

This pose is great at strengthening and toning the whole body as well as improving alignment and balance.

Stand straight with your feet together. Spread your toes out wide apart and make sure you distribute your weight evenly over both feet. Using your muscles around your knees and thighs, pull your kneecaps up, move your thighs back and tuck your tailbone in. Keep your arms straight by your side, palms facing in. Pull back your shoulder blades and lift your chest, keeping your neck and shoulders relaxed. Look straight ahead. Hold for 1–2 minutes.

Be conscious in this pose and don't just relax. Activate every part of your body, from your feet all the way up to your head.

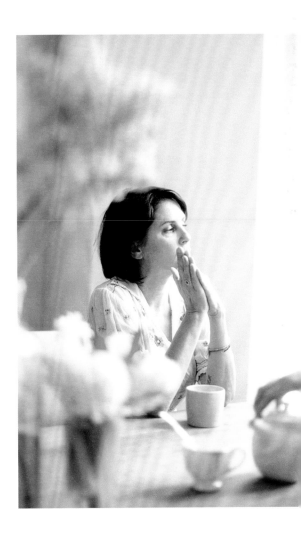

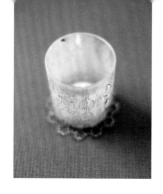

yoga for

ANGER

A twist can be beneficial for wringing out anger because anger is often held in our inner organs, especially the liver. One of its roles is to transform hormones released during negative emotional states, so they can be eliminated from the body. If the liver is not functioning properly then it is unable to release the hormones. This causes the body to heat up and negative states such as anger are prolonged.

Ardha Matsyendrasana (Half spinal twist)
The half spinal twist is very beneficial for both the liver and spleen. When you inhale you are breathing fresh new life and then letting everything that is stale and old be washed away by the exhalation.

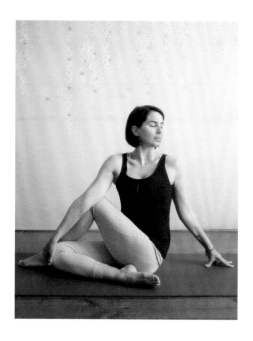

Sit on the floor, with your legs straight in front of you. Now bend both your knees and put your feet flat on the floor.

Slide your right foot under your left leg, all the way to the outside of your left hip. Gently lay the right side of your leg on the floor.

Take your left foot and step it over the right leg. Stand it on the floor beside your right hip. Your left knee should be pointing to the ceiling. Exhale and half twist your spine towards your left thigh.
Put your left hand behind you on the floor by your left buttock.

Put your right upper arm on the outside of your left thigh near the knee.

Keep your tailbone lengthened and make sure your left foot stays firmly in contact with the floor.

Turn your head in the direction of the twist, so towards the left.

With every inhalation lift your chest a little more through the sternum and then twist deeper as you exhale. Stay in this position for about 30 seconds to 1 minute and then repeat on the other side.

Sarvang Asana (Basic shoulder stand)
This is another pose that is beneficial at reducing stress and getting rid of any feelings of anger. It helps to increase the blood flow to the upper body especially the neck, shoulders and head. It has lots of other benefits including relieving allergies, helping with asthma, stimulating your thyroid and it can also calm your nervous system.

With this exercise you need to be especially precise, and mindful of your back and your neck so that there is no risk of injury.

Lie on the floor with your legs together. Put your arms close to your body, palms facing up. Make sure you press your head onto the floor and your shoulders and arms are rooted.

Exhale and swing your legs over your head lifting your hips. Elongate your body as long as possible and support your hips with your hands. Be aware of your foundation, keeping the weight distributed mainly on the elbows, then your shoulders and then your head. If you are comfortable and you feel rooted, hold the position for ten breaths. Once you have achieved this, slowly come down, keeping your weight on your hands to protect your back and neck.

IN SOME FORMS OF YOGA, IT IS ADVISED TO USE A ROLLED-UP BLANKET THAT IS PLACED UNDER THE EDGE OF YOUR SHOULDERS AND NOT UNDER YOUR HEAD AND NECK. THIS CREATES MORE SPACE, EASING PRESSURE ON YOUR NECK.

Shavasana (The corpse pose)
As the name suggests, this pose requires you to be as still as a corpse. To get the full benefit you need to clear your mind of any thoughts and breathe deeply. This pose (my favourite!) is amazing at relaxing your entire body.

Lie on your back with your legs slightly apart. Put your arms beside your body with the palms facing upwards. Close your eyes and release any tension from your face, making sure your jaw isn't clenched. Start to visualise every part of your body relaxing, beginning with your feet then your legs, organs, arms and continue up to your head.

You need to spend 5–15 minutes practising Shavasana so that you fully relax your body.

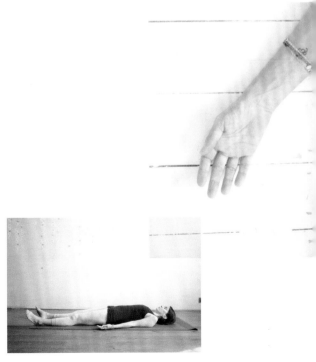

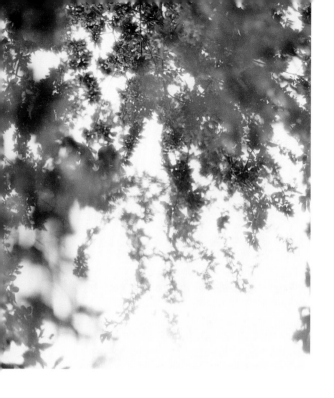

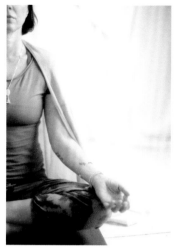

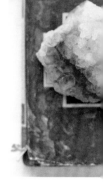

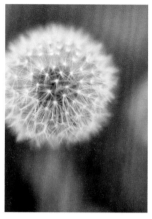

MEDITATION

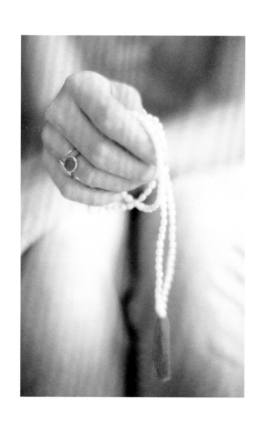

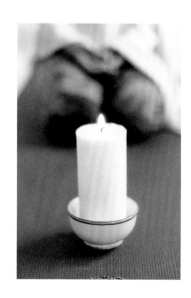

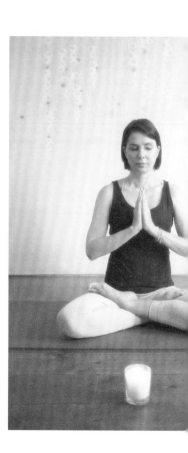

Meditation is something I struggled with right from the beginning. I just didn't get it! I really felt that I was kind of faking it and I just didn't understand what it actually achieved. But I persevered and did many courses with different people, from gong meditation (somebody plays on a huge gong to create really positive vibrations that wash through your body and cleanse your mind) to transcendental meditation and many others. There are many kinds of meditation and you have to really find the type that works for you.

Science has now proved that deep relaxation changes the genetic level of our bodies. One Harvard study found the disease-fighting genes increasing in activity after relaxation practices. Relaxation is a state of rest and physical renewal. It boosts your nervous system by activating the parasympathetic nervous system, causing the body to feel more relaxed. You will have improved digestion, better memory, a stronger immune system, you will find yourself more emotionally balanced, with lower blood pressure and a reduction in those cancer-causing free radicals. This state also decreases the mental and physical ageing process, improves PMS and decreases the chances of contracting heart disease.

Meditation is a state of thoughtless awareness; it is effortless. The benefits of meditation are endless, and it can be practised anywhere at any time for free.

There are many styles of meditation practice and it may take you a few tries at different approaches until you find one that suits you. I would suggest you meditate for 10–20 minutes daily and commit to practising for 21 days to give yourself the best chance to experience the benefits. Remember some days will be easier than others but you will still be benefiting.

FOLLOWING
THE BREATH

As the name suggests, this form of meditation focuses on your breath. Make no effort to control the breath, just observe its rhythm with no judgement. Some breaths will be deep, and some shallow. Just concentrate your mind on your breathing: every time you notice yourself in thought, gently bring your attention back to the breath.

Sit upright with your spine straight. You can either kneel, cross your legs or sit on a chair with your feet on the floor. Place your hands, palms turned upwards, on your thighs or knees.

Inhale and exhale, slowly and deeply, three times. Focus on relaxing your body as you breathe out. Your eyes can be open or closed; I prefer to close them.

Then just allow your breath to come in of its own accord: make no attempt to control it. Simply observe your breath, flowing in, and flowing out. If any thoughts come, just notice them and let them go, and return your attention to your breath.

Feel the air flow effortlessly in through your nostrils and into your abdomen. Feel your abdomen rise on the inhalation then fall again as the breath flows out.

Sometimes people like to concentrate on the whole breath, but you may find it easier just to focus on the breath's movement through your nose, or in your abdomen or maybe in your diaphragm, whatever works best for you.

JUST CONCENTRATE YOUR MIND ON YOUR BREATHING: EVERY TIME YOU NOTICE YOURSELF IN THOUGHT, GENTLY BRING YOUR ATTENTION BACK TO YOUR BREATH.

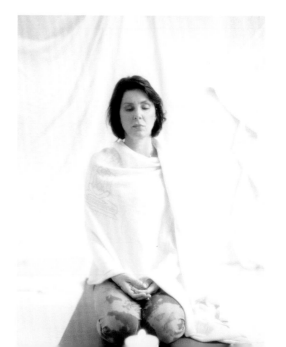

MANTRA MEDITATION

During a mantra meditation you mentally repeat a calming word, sound or mantra that will take you away from all your busy thoughts. Again your mind will wander and when you notice that it has, just gently bring your attention back to your mantra.

There is no right or wrong way to do this. Just remember to relax and let the mantra effortlessly fill your mind. Some days my mind is so busy that I barely remember to come back to my mantra but even so I still feel and receive the benefits.

You begin in an upright seated position just as you did with the previous meditation exercise.

Inhale and exhale deeply three times. Instead of focusing on the breath, replace the awareness with mentally repeating your mantra.

A few popular mantras are:
Omlaum (it is, will be, to become)
Love
Ham-Sah (a Hindu variant meaning I am he/that)
I am that I am
Om Mani Padme Hum (hail the jewel in the lotus)

Another form of mantra meditation is transcendental meditation, or TM, where the teacher provides you with a mantra. There are many places that teach TM: I can highly recommend the David Lynch Foundation as being very reputable and a good place to learn.

MINDFUL MEDITATION

During mindful meditation you expand your awareness of the present moment – your focus is entirely based on what you are experiencing at that point in time.

Mindful meditation can be practised whether you are sitting or moving around. Your focus could be on a thought, or your breath, or the sensation of your hands on your legs or your feet on the floor. It seems quite simple but even the act of sitting and focusing on one thing can bring you back into the now and ease you into a light meditation.

Alternatively you can practise mindful meditation as you go about your everyday business, for example while washing up, cooking, shopping, or walking down the street. The reason this works is we can use these normal daily activities as our focus. We become mindful of our experiences, keeping our awareness involved. I prefer walking meditation, which I use daily while walking to the station on my way to work.

Unlike the other forms of meditation, you keep your eyes open during this meditation. There is a focus and an awareness that sometimes gets ignored if we don't actively practise mindful meditation. This might be the sounds of nature, other people, cars or machines.

Meditating while your body is in motion seems for most people to be easier compared to when you are sitting still. This is because a lot of people don't have the patience to sit still and you can feel uncomfortable sitting still for a long time.

This meditation can be an intense experience and can also bring enjoyment. As long as you are aware of yourself, you are being mindful. Again there is no need to change anything or to judge. Just observe whatever is happening, your thoughts, feelings or sensations. It is simply about bringing your attention into the moment, focusing your awareness fully on what you are doing.

CANDLE MEDITATION

This form of meditation can lead you into an intense meditation that will bring you serenity, calmness and improve your concentration. In this hypnotic state, the mind settles and you can focus your attention on no topic at all and allow your mind to become completely quiet.

You want your environment to be comfortable before you begin this technique – make sure you are warm and the lights are dimmed.

Place a burning candle that is at eye level when you adopt an upright seated position.

Deeply inhale and exhale three times.

Focus your attention on the candle flame, watching with ease how it flickers. Sit for a while like this and then in your own time close your eyes.

Now focus your attention on your mind's eye or third eye, which is situated on the bridge of your nose between your eyebrows. You will most likely see the imprint and image of the flickering flame in your imagination. If for any reason you don't, reopen your eyes and watch the burning flame until when you close your eyes again you have the image of the flame imprinted in your mind.

Gently observe the image in your mind's eye until it fades away, then open your eyes again and repeat. As before, there is no right or wrong way to do this; it is meant to be relaxing and effortless. Repeat this exercise for 10–20 minutes.

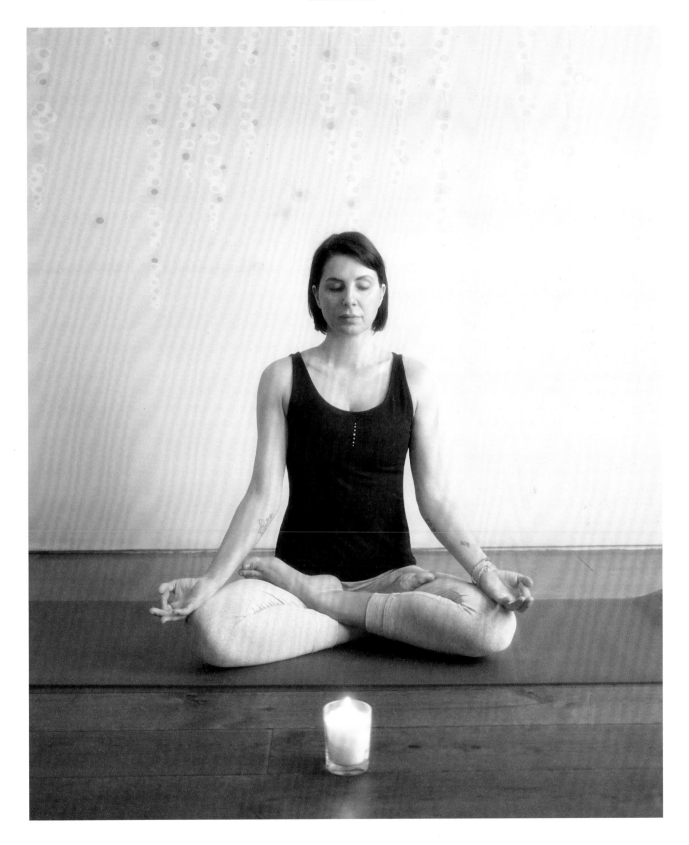

ORGANISING YOUR DAY

how to keep on track & stay positive

For all of us women there is a lot to do within a day. We all have very busy lives and we are constantly multi-tasking. In my case having four kids, three businesses, a need to exercise, run my home, my life, kids' lives, dogs' lives, wanting to eat healthily and so on … it can all become really stressful. And yes, sometimes my regime completely falls apart. I eat the wrong food, drink too much and some days I just don't feel motivated to exercise. But nobody is perfect and when you feel like this you just have to draw a line under that day and start again. Well, that's what I do! But we have to keep on going and moderate our lives rather than being judgemental and self-critical.

Through everything you do, you still have to love yourself. I always tell myself that provided I am good 95 per cent of the time, for the other 5 per cent I can live my life feeling less pressurised and constrained, and that way ultimately I can be happy, as I am not under such scrutiny. After all, it is so important to live life to the full. A friend said to me once, 'Sadie, you have got to start living. Stop worrying!' If you start considering how many summers you have left when you will be physically fit enough or adventurous enough to jump off the side of a boat, it gives you the impetus to utilise your time more fully and actually go for it and be daring!

With so much to think about there are several strategies to help you put yourself under less pressure, not least being organised and managing your time carefully – especially if you have a very full day ahead of you. When I've got a busy day ahead and I know I won't have time to get food I put a couple of sachets of miso soup and a pack of almonds in my handbag for snacking on. Then I won't get hungry and reach for a chocolate bar. And even though making lists, schedules and keeping diaries may seem a little clinical, they do help you feel in control and confident that you're getting everything done, which keeps your mind at peace.

I like to try to make the first few hours after I wake as smooth as possible because if that happens then the rest of the day tends to work out too. Preparing

I LIKE TO TRY TO MAKE THE FIRST
FEW HOURS AFTER I WAKE AS SMOOTH
AS POSSIBLE BECAUSE IF THAT
HAPPENS THEN THE REST OF THE DAY
TENDS TO WORK OUT TOO.

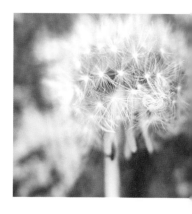

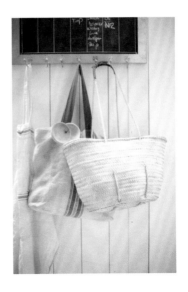

breakfast, doing the school run and getting to work can all become a lot easier if we follow a few simple steps and start the day focused, grounded and unstressed. Of course, if you can include a walking meditation when you are walking to work, returning from school or taking your dogs to the park, you ground yourself and start the day positive and calm. While I walk my dogs, I try to think of as many positive thoughts as possible. If a negative thought comes into my mind I replace it with a positive. The more you do this the more your mind has positive thoughts. Harbouring resentments is not good for anyone, so if I am consumed with resentment towards somebody or something I try my hardest to alleviate this. A friend of mine gave me a tip for times when my mind is full of resentful thoughts about one person or some intense situation. She suggested I visualise shrinking the thought or image in question, turning it into black and white and sending it to another part of the world. I tried this and it really works; it gives the resentment less importance.

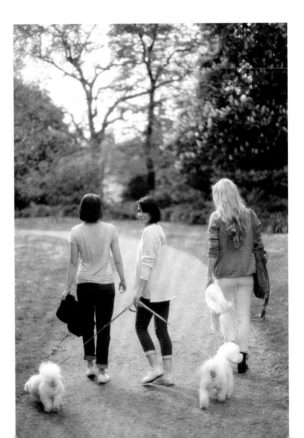

my morning

ROUTINE

I start my day with oil swilling, which is also called oil pulling. I swill a small spoonful of unrefined good-quality oil (I use coconut) all around my mouth, like you would with a mouthwash but with none of the chemicals those products contain. Oil swilling attracts and removes bacteria, toxins and parasites that live in your mouth or lymph system, and also pulls any congestion and mucus from your throat and loosens up your sinuses. With the help of your saliva, all these unwanted things bind with the oil, ready to be spat out. The process also helps to re-mineralise your teeth and strengthen your gums by thoroughly cleansing the mouth area.

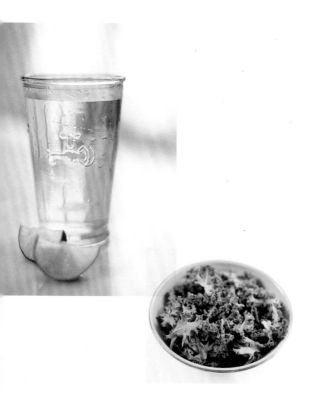

While I am swilling I do some gentle stretches like the Downward Facing Dog (see page 132) or I kneel in Child's Pose (see page 136) or I just kneel with my big toes together and my bottom on my heels. I exhale and place my forehead on the floor, swilling the whole time. In this position I will take many breaths, breathing into my spine, creating space. After just a few minutes it is amazing how much my spine has lengthened. Another simple exercise to warm up and extend the spine is to sit cross legged and rotate from the hips. Firstly clockwise, then reverse circles anticlockwise, 5 one way and 5 the other, with your hands on your knees pressing down, pushing your torso in a circle.

Any of these exercises allows me to create some space in my body, aligning my spine and lengthening my breath. I finish with a short meditation, usually in Lotus position (Padmasana), which means sitting cross-legged. To perfect this pose each foot is placed on the opposite thigh, keeping the knee joint as close as possible to the floor while rotating your hip joints.

My routine takes about 20 minutes, which is enough time to swill. Once I have finished the oil swilling, I spit the oil into a tissue and put it in the bin to avoid any issues with blocking toilets or sinks. Then, I swish out my mouth a few times with clean water.

After a night's sleep your body can become quite acidic. To counteract this I prepare myself a cup of warm water and squeeze the juice of a lemon or half a lemon (or lime) into it; this restores my body to a more alkaline state. Even though lemon tastes very bitter and tart, it is in fact alkaline and not acidic. Another good tip to alkalise the body in the morning is to add a tablespoon of apple cider vinegar to a glass of water. The whole acid/alkaline food topic is very interesting and I try to follow it as closely as I can (see opposite).

GREEN POWER
SMOOTHIE

The last part of my morning routine is to make a power smoothie. This one, invented by my sister Jade, will set you up for the whole day!

Juicing and drinking smoothies is quite controversial at the moment. My advice is to eat a healthy diet and enjoy juicing and green smoothies from time to time. Supplementing juicing and smoothies for meals is not a good idea.

1 banana
1 small sachet acai pulp
1 handful frozen berries
2 tablespoons protein powder
1 handful spinach or kale
2 teaspoons super green mix
  (spirulina, wheat grass and
  barley grass)
600ml almond milk
1 teaspoon bee pollen

Put everything apart from the bee pollen into a blender and blitz for about 45 seconds. Add more almond milk if you prefer a thinner consistency. Pour into a glass and sprinkle the bee pollen on top – it gives the smoothie a lovely little crunch and tastes delicious!

Tips to counter too much acid in the body:

Drink plenty of water – 3 litres a day is best. Make sure it is filtered.

Have a big salad once a day, which includes green leafy vegetables such as kale, spinach, broccoli, asparagus and parsley.

Use black pepper on anything savoury.

Snack on pumpkin seeds or add them to salads.

Swap your table salt for Himalayan or sea salt.

Drink ginger tea as it is very alkalising.

Swap balsamic vinegar for apple cider vinegar.

Squeeze lemon or lime juice on salads or in your herbal teas.

Reduce stress – it plays a big role on the pH of your body and whether it is acidic or alkaline.

FENG SHUI

It doesn't require a lot of effort or investment to organise your home along Feng Shui principles and the benefits can be immediate. You should enjoy bringing positive energy into your home and feel a lot happier and healthier for it.

Steps to Remove Negative Energy

Decluttering removes negative energy and frees space to bring new life and positive forces into your home.

1) Start by opening windows/doors to allow the air to flow freely. Draw back the curtains and let the light shine in.

2) Clear out all your clutter, as this will be blocking your good energy and fortune. Typical areas where we allow clutter to accumulate are behind doors, on tops of wardrobes and under beds.

3) Give your home a thorough clean from top to bottom. Hopefully, it will be less of a mammoth task now that you have dealt with those junk spots.

4) Sound is a very effective and instant way to clear the energy in any space. Start by walking around your home clapping; this will break up any stagnant or blocked energy, allowing it to flow freely. Alternatively, walk around your home ringing a bell or chanting or singing. Singing clears and uplifts the energy of your home, as does playing music.

Rebalancing Your Home

Feng Shui uses the four elements of Fire, Water, Earth and Air to bring balance and harmony into a space.

Fire

Fire has been used for purification since ancient times. Churches, mosques, synagogues and temples all use fire in their religious and sacred rituals. In your home cleansing with fire is as simple as lighting a candle. Whenever I light a candle I put my intention forward – be it a need to bring peace and well-being or a more specific intention such as to attract a mate or get a job. Then I place it in the appropriate area – for example, if I am having problems with my finances, I place the candle in my Fortunate Blessings Area.

Water

Water is the symbol of harmony. For best results, use water from a natural spring or waterfall, or water from an unpolluted river or stream. Bless the water by holding your hands over the bowl while you either pray or chant, all the while focusing on your intentions. Then use the blessed water to purify your home, sprinkling it wherever you feel inclined. I put the water into a spray bottle and walk around spraying the entire space.

Earth

Salt is a powerful means of purification and is universally renowned for its healing properties. It is also said to absorb negativity. When I space clear I like to put either a bowl of salt in every room, or a line of salt across every doorway. Leave the salt for 24 hours, by which time it should have absorbed all the negativity.

Air

Burning incense is one of the most readily available and popular ways of purifying the air. You can also burn essential oils in an oil burner.

Electromagnetic fields

Electromagnetic fields, or EMFs, are environmental pollution. EMFs are the fields created by electrical wiring, satellite dishes, microwaves, televisions and all the technical devices most of us have in our homes. Ways in which you can reduce the severity of EMFs include turning off all appliances at the mains and pulling out the plugs. Placing plants and crystals near or on electrical equipment helps to lessen the EMFs.

Crystals

Crystals are powerful Feng Shui aids that can be placed in an appropriate area of your home to absorb negative energy and promote healing. There are many books and websites on the properties of crystals: rose quartz, for example, is the crystal of love; amethyst is thought to promote peace and tranquillity. I place an amethyst crystal under my bed to encourage a peaceful night's sleep.

Crystals that help alleviate and block geopathic and environmental stress are brown jasper, amazonite, amethyst, diamonds (worn as earrings are very effective against the rays that are emitted by mobile phones), fluorite, larimar, obsidian and smoky quartz. Placing any of these crystals by your computer, microwave or television, along with plants such as peace lilies, spider plants, and Chinese evergreens can help clear geopathic stress and cleanse the air.

Flowers

Flowers are used for their colour and beauty to enhance and uplift any space. They can also be used alongside plants in specific areas to raise the energy levels. Always use fresh flowers and keep the water clear.

EMBRACING FENG SHUI IS A FUN AND POSITIVE EXPERIENCE THAT WILL ALLOW GOOD TO FLOW INTO YOUR LIFE.

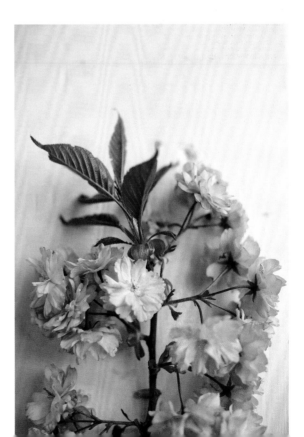

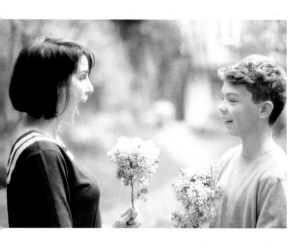

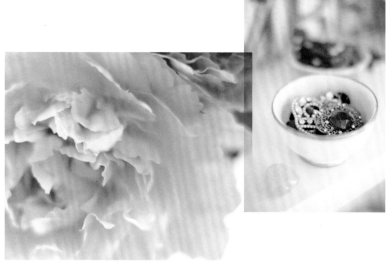

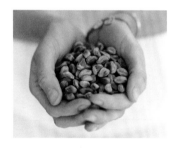

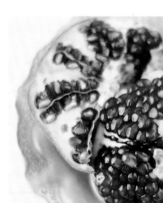

HEALTH

&

BEAUTY

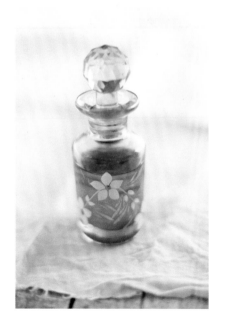

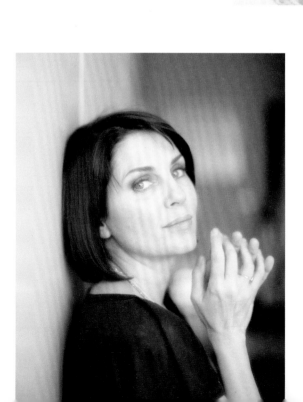

For ultimate health and beauty, I believe we should try and have as much of a naturalistic approach as possible. When I see someone radiating both health and beauty from inside and out it is the most beautiful and simple thing. It is not a daunting or complicated process, but one where you consider different factors and try to look at the whole approach to health rather than just trying to find a cream that will make your skin look better on the outside.

When you see a supple, lean body, it usually shows a person who eats well and moderately and who exercises so they are agile and energised.

In my next section, I give some simple and holistic ideas on how to achieve glowing skin, hair care, how to radiate health and some simple tips that you can add to your daily routine to make you feel at your best. There are some face packs, body soaks and other treats that I love using when I need that extra bit of nourishment. There are also a few quick tips to add to your daily routine that I have found to be very beneficial and make me feel at my best.

It doesn't have to be complicated but to have general wellbeing, health, happiness and beauty, you need to address it from all areas: your diet, fresh air, fresh, healthy food, body-brushing, some form of exercise, lots of water, lots of sleep and making sure you have peace of mind. If you do all of these you will be able to achieve your optimum in both health and beauty.

love your

SKIN & HAIR

It's entirely possible to spend a small fortune on skin and haircare products, but there are lots of natural ingredients you will have in your home that will do amazing things for your appearance at a fraction of the cost.

Of course, plenty of fresh fruit and vegetables in your daily diet is good for your appearance, but directly applying natural ingredients to your skin and hair will also help. Here are some of my favourite natural remedies:

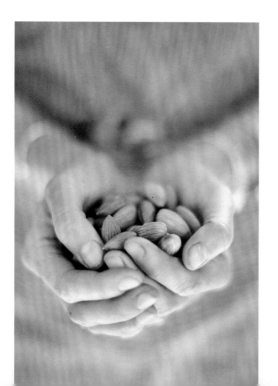

Almond oil

This is an incredible source of vitamins A, B and E, all of which are great for your skin's health. Almond oil helps in maintaining the moisture levels of your skin and gets absorbed really quickly without blocking your pores. It is particularly useful if you have extremely dry, sensitive or irritated skin.

Avocado

This wonder fruit is rich in monounsaturated oils, which are easily absorbed into the skin. Avocados also contain vitamin E, one of the best ingredients for dry skin, and they plump your skin with lots of moisturising benefits.

Banana

This tasty fruit contains significant amounts of vitamin C and B6, both of which play vital roles in maintaining the elasticity of the skin, as well as Vitamin A. Mashed banana's a great natural moisturiser that helps repair damaged, dull and dry skin.

Eggs

Eggs too help with the repair of skin tissue. Egg white is great for generally toning the skin and closing pores and the yolk acts as a natural moisturiser. The lutein contained in egg yolk is immensely good at keeping your skin elastic and hydrated.

Beaten egg makes a great conditioner for dry and brittle hair – just apply it to damp hair, leave for 20 minutes then rinse off with warm water.

Goat's milk

Goat's milk contains precious minerals like selenium and is packed full of vitamins, particularly A, the most important vitamin for skin. As with other milks, goat's milk contains lactic acid, an alpha hydroxy acid (AHA) that can gently slough off dead skin cells and help to hydrate and brighten the skin. Goat's milk is an extremely useful beauty ingredient because it is rich in essential fatty acids and triglycerides. The pH of those essential fatty acids is similar to that of humans, so it is less likely to irritate and is easily absorbed by your skin.

Honey

This delicious sweetener is another natural moisturiser that works wonders on dry skin. It also has many antiseptic qualities, which can be very beneficial to people with oily skin that is prone to breakouts. Applied directly to the skin honey leaves a very soft, satiny feel.

Lemon

Lemon juice is a natural antiseptic so it is a great ingredient to apply to your skin and hair. It is a cooling agent that helps with skin problems such as sunburn, insect stings, acne and eczma. It also acts as an anti-ageing remedy and can remove wrinkles by contributing to collagen production.

Lemon juice can also be used on your hair to treat problems like dandruff and acts as a stimulant if you find your hair is falling out. A tablespoon of lemon juice applied directly to washed, towel-dried hair can give it real shine, and it is great for blonde hair that needs a little boost.

Oats

Oats contain vitamin E, which is one of the antioxidant vitamins that can help counteract the damaging effect of free radicals in the skin. Oats are very soothing, gently exfoliating and they help to lighten the skin.

Sugar

Sugar is a natural humectant, meaning it absorbs moisture from the environment so, when you apply sugar to your skin, it actually helps to hydrate it and keep moisture within. It is also a natural source of glycolic acid, another alpha hydroxy acid (AHA) that penetrates the skin and breaks down the 'glue' that bonds skin cells, encouraging the cell regeneration that gives you fresher, younger-looking skin. Sugar makes a great exfoliant when added to other ingredients; you can choose granulated, brown or caster sugar depending on how deep you want to scrub (see page 156).

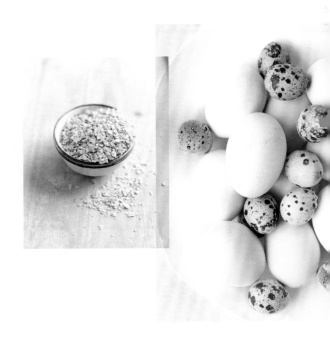

FACE PACKS & BODY SCRUBS

Avocado face pack

Avocado is wonderful for adding moisture to tired or dry skin thanks to the vitamin E and monounsaturated oils it contains. Simply mash the flesh of 1 ripe avocado in a bowl and apply to your face and neck. Leave for 30 minutes and then wipe off using cotton wool dipped in warm water.

For combination skin

Simply add 1 beaten egg yolk to the mashed avocado. Apply to the face and leave for 30 minutes then remove with damp cotton wool.

For tired, ageing skin

Add 1 tablespoon of honey and 1 beaten egg yolk to the mashed avocado and mix to a smooth creamy texture. Apply to the face and leave for 30 minutes, then remove with damp cotton wool.

Honey and banana face pack

Try using this if your skin feels dehydrated – honey and banana are both extremely moisturising. Mash 1 small ripe banana in a bowl until it's a smooth creamy paste. Stir in 25g oatmeal and 1 teaspoon of runny honey. Apply to the face and leave for 15–20 minutes then remove with damp cotton wool.

Lemon cleanser

Lemon juice acts as an antibacterial agent, so it will help with oily skin, breakouts and also balances the pH of the skin. The egg white tightens and tones the skin.

Mix together 1 teaspoon of freshly squeezed lemon juice and 1 stiffly beaten egg white and apply to your face. Leave for about 10 minutes and then wash off in warm water or with rose water.

Sugar scrub

Sugar has an antibacterial as well as an exfoliating effect on the skin, so this scrub is really beneficial for oily or spotty skin. Choose from caster, granulated or Demerara sugar, depending on how deep you want to scrub. I recommend Demerara or granulated for the body and caster sugar for the face and neck. Mix 1 teaspoon sugar with a few drops of hot water in your hands and gently massage into your skin. Rinse off with cool water and pat dry with a towel.

Coconut and rose body scrub

Try using this scrub on your body while you're waiting for your bath to fill up. It works so well at exfoliating and hydrating skin. Soothing coconut oil combined with sugar will scrape off dead skin cells and clean blocked pores without irritating your skin. The oil will leave the skin soft, even and help close your pores. The sugar is antibacterial, so great for dealing with breakouts.

60ml coconut oil
60g granulated sugar
10 drops rose essential oil

Mix the ingredients together in a bowl. Take some of the mixture and gently rub over your body paying particular attention to any hard areas of skin on your elbows, knees and heels. Once you have rubbed it all over, get into your bath and rinse it off. The coconut oil and sugar will dissolve into the bath and make it smell amazing! Soak for as long as you like.

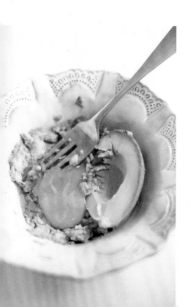

BATH SOAKS

Retreating to a warm bath can work miracles on skin problems, aching joints and sore muscles and is generally therapeutic after a hectic or stressful day. Adding everyday ingredients such as sea salt and tea or essential oils such as lavender or rose to the water will soothe specific ailments.

Detox bath

Try this soak to help with skin irritations, boost your magnesium levels or for a great detoxifying bath after a stressful day at work.

60g sea salt or Himalayan salt
60g Epsom salts
60g bicarbonate of soda
80g apple cider vinegar
10 drops essential oil, e.g. lavender, peppermint, rose

Put the salts and bicarbonate of soda into a heatproof jug. Add 150ml of boiling water and allow the salts to dissolve. Fill the bath with warm/hot water and add the apple cider vinegar and the essential oils. Lastly add the salts to the bath.

Soak in the bath for about 30 minutes. This is a detoxifying bath and you may feel lightheaded when you get out, so do be careful.

Milky bath

This bath soak leaves your skin feeling silky smooth due to the lactic acid in the milk, which hydrates the skin and helps with exfoliation.

Warm 500ml goat's milk in a pan and add to your hot bath. Soak in the bath for around 20–30 minutes. You can add 10 drops of your favourite essential oil to help you relax even more.

A bath full of tea!

This bath soak is so easy to do. Simply brew 3–4 large cups of strong hot tea and add them to your bath. Try different types of teas for different effects. Here are a few of my personal favourites to choose from but feel free to experiment with any tea you like:

English breakfast tea
This is good for itchy skin as the blend contains high levels of tannins that have both anti-inflammatory and anti-viral effects.

Chamomile tea
Chamomile has a calming effect on the body so this is a relaxing and soothing bath. Perfect at bedtime, it is also beneficial for skin conditions like eczema and chicken pox, common swellings or infection.

Green tea
The B vitamins in green tea can make you feel happier and lift your spirits, leaving you feeling uplifted and energised. Green tea is also full of antioxidants polyphenols, theanine and tannin that have powerful effects on the body, soothing sore muscles, open wounds, rashes, cold sores, and many more.

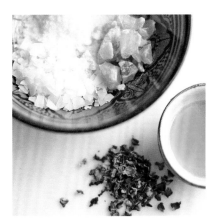

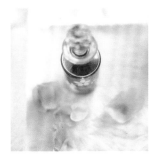

FACE & NECK
EXERCISES

It's so important to keep the facial muscles toned and supple. Facial exercises keep your skin looking younger and help reduce lines. All of these can be done when you're waiting for a bus, you've stopped at a red light or are walking in the park.

Skin can be very forgiving. Of course you can't reverse the ageing process completely but by stimulating blood circulation you can tighten and stimulate tone the natural contours of your face. We go to the gym and work out our bodies, so why not do the same for our faces? With regular exercises, you will see a big change, so give it a go.

Eyes

Our eyes can be one of the first places to show signs of ageing. To keep them toned and reduce sagging muscles and crow's feet, try these yoga facial exercises. They will also strengthen your eyes.

Take a deep breath in and keep your head in its normal position. Without moving your head, look up as high as you can. Hold the pose for 5–10 seconds.

Now look downwards and hold for 5–10 seconds.

Look up to the top right corner and hold this pose for 5–10 seconds.

Next, look up to the top left corner and hold for 5–10 seconds.

Then start rotating your eyes in a clockwise motion, trying to look as far as you can to the corners, top and bottom. Do this a few times and then repeat in an anticlockwise direction.

BY STIMULATING BLOOD CIRCULATION
YOU CAN TIGHTEN AND TONE THE NATURAL
CONTOURS OF YOUR FACE.

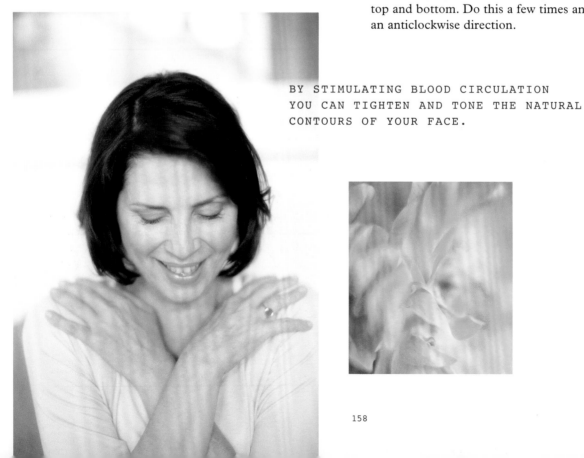

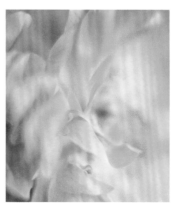

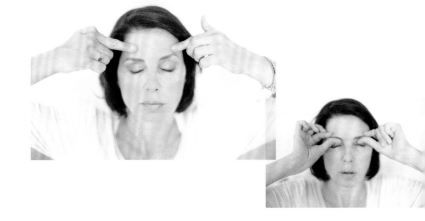

Mouth

We use our mouths to eat, drink, talk, sing and smile. With time they can lose tone and start to droop at the corners making us look unhappy. By doing the exercises below you will strengthen the muscles around your lips and prevent drooping. Do these exercises every day to put the smile back on your face!

Pretend you are kissing the air: pucker your lips as tightly as you can and blow 10 kisses.

With your mouth closed, use your tongue to feel all around the outside of your top teeth. Start with the molars at the back and move your tongue all the way to the other side and then repeat with the bottom teeth. Keep moving your tongue round in this circular movement and then go the other way. Do this 10–15 times.

Keeping your lips together, blow out the right cheek to make a balloon shape and hold for a few seconds. Then do the same with your left cheek and repeat 20 times. Then blow out both cheeks at the same time and slowly release the air. This works on reducing laughter lines by toning the facial muscles around this area.

Use your thumbs and index fingers to hold your upper lip. Your thumbnail will touch the upper gums. Totally relax and gently pull your lip downwards. Move along the whole lip and repeat 5 times. This will help with any lines across the top of the lip.

Forehead

We use our forehead for lots of expressions and, with time, lines begin to appear, especially if we frown a lot! By releasing the tension in these muscles, we create better blood flow and allow the muscles to relax and go back to their normal position.

To get rid of these lines, use your fingertips to make circular movements around the top of your scalp. Reducing tension here helps the forehead. Do this for a couple of minutes.

Take the palm of your hand and press it against your forehead. Keeping your hand in that position, try to move your head downwards. This will pull your forehead up and act as a lifting technique. Repeat this process 5 times.

Place your thumbs on your temples and both index fingers in the centre of the top of your forehead. Pull upwards and you should feel your whole forehead lifting upwards. Hold it for 5 seconds and then repeat the action 5–10 times.

Eyebrows

These exercises release the tension around the eyebrows and are really good at easing tension and headaches. They help to reduce frown lines and give the eyes a more lifted appearance.

Put your thumbs on either side of the top of your nose where your eyebrows start. Using your index fingers and thumbs, pinch the fleshy part around the eyebrows and use circular movements all the way along to massage and release the muscle. You can increase the pressure a little bit each time.

Sweep your index fingers along the eyebrows starting from the bridge of your nose and ending at your temples. You can increase the pressure each time – it should feel like a big release of pressure.

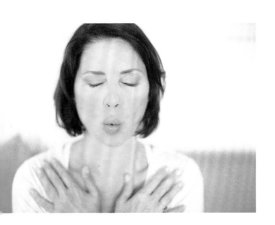

FACE & NECK
EXERCISES

Neck

The skin around our necks is very fine and is one of the first places where we notice signs of ageing. These techniques will really help to strengthen the muscles of your jaw as well as the platysma, the band of muscle that surrounds your collarbone and upper chest.

Lift your head upwards, looking at the sky, to lengthen your neck. Using the back of both hands, sweep upwards from the bottom of your neck all the way to the chin. Continue the action for 30 seconds.

Tensing all the muscles in your neck, slowly move your head from right to left. Repeat 10 times, alternating the direction each time. This will tone all the muscles in your neck and stop the skin from sagging.

Look straight ahead and tense all the muscles in your neck. Keep looking to the same point and stick your neck forwards but not downwards. Then bring it back to the normal position. Repeat 10 times.

To finish

Place your index fingers either side of the bridge of your nose and make small circular movements to the bottom of your nose around your nostrils. This especially helps to clear nasal congestion and aids lymphatic drainage.

Using your thumbs and index fingers, pinch and pluck the skin all over your face. This increases the blood flow and circulation to the face and is the perfect way to end the exercises.

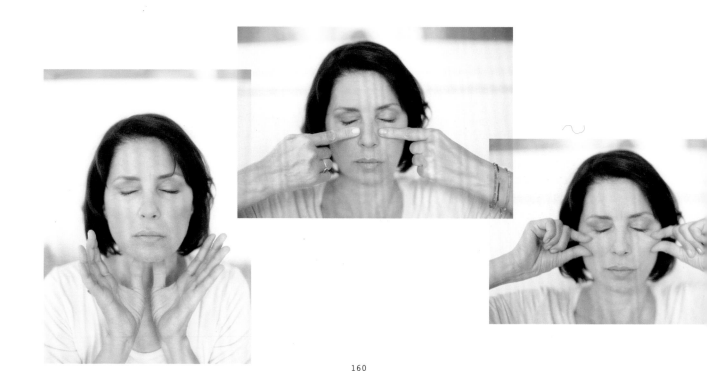

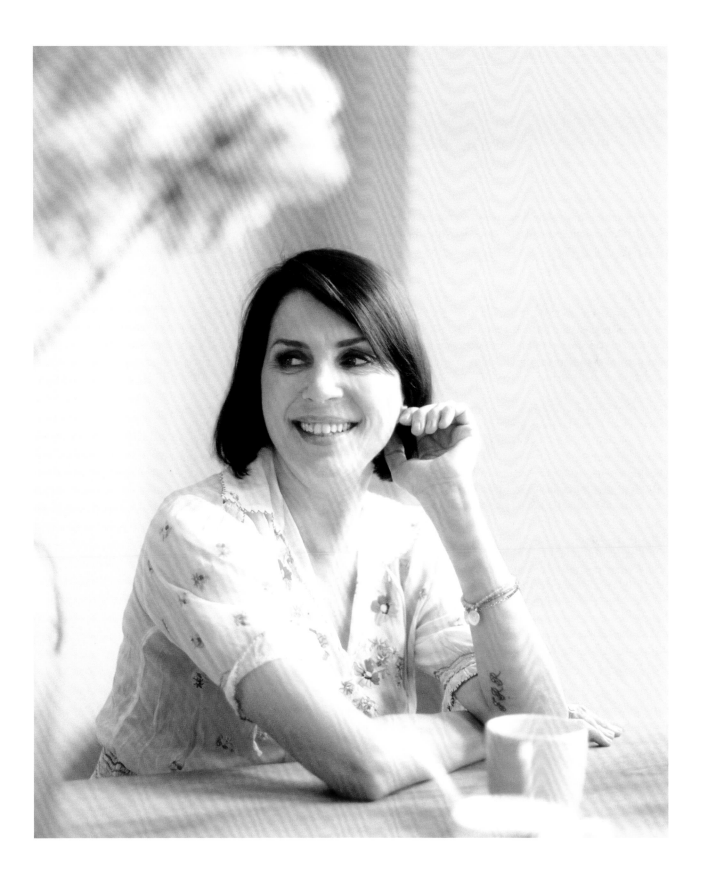

BODY BRUSHING

I couldn't live without...

REFLEXOLOGY

Body brushing has really done wonders for me; since I have been doing it every day I have seen huge benefits. The tone of my skin has changed, muscle definition has increased, cellulite has disappeared, my metabolism has improved and literally I feel more alive. It can be done on dry or wet skin, either just before you shower or while you are in it. Body brushing on dry skin has been shown to be the better: done on a daily basis it can provide a number of benefits such as improving the circulation, stimulating lymph drainage and stimulating hormones as well as firming the skin.

Body brushes are easily bought from a chemist or health store. They typically have short, firm bristles – look for one made with natural not synthetic bristles and a long-handle to make it easy to brush all your body. Body brushing works in a number of ways. By improving vascular blood circulation and lymph drainage, it encourages the discharge of metabolic waste, hence the body can run more effectively. It also helps with the nervous system by stimulating the nerve endings so they work better. It increases the absorption of nutrients by eliminating clogged pores and it also helps shift cellulite, which is a toxic material that accumulates in fat cells.

Start body brushing first thing in the morning before you have your shower. I prefer to brush in a warm shower on wet skin. I brush for 5–10 minutes and afterwards take a cold shower. I strongly advise you to do this – you will notice such a difference. Take your brush and (gently at first) brush in long strokes starting from your feet and always working upwards towards your heart. Once you have brushed all the way up to your shoulders, start brushing from your hands towards your shoulders with long sweeping strokes. Overlap the strokes and repeat over the same section 2–3 times. Don't brush over any broken skin or sensitive areas.

Reflexology makes you feel calm and grounded and sorts out many ailments you may have, including headaches, digestive problems, insomnia and stress. It works by stimulating, massaging and applying pressure to different points in your feet or hands (or sometimes ears) in order to stimulate energy flow through the body and promote self-healing.

Reflexologists believe that the body is divided into ten vertical zones or channels, five on the left and five on the right. Each zone runs from the head down to the reflex areas on the feet and hands. By applying pressure to these reflex points you can stimulate the energy flow through the corresponding body part and release an energy block in any part of the zone.

It brings about a deep relaxation and can help return the body to its natural state. It may help with conditions including headaches, digestive problems, insomnia and stress.

REFLEXOLOGY WORKS BY STIMULATING ENERGY FLOW THROUGH THE BODY TO PROMOTE SELF-HEALING.

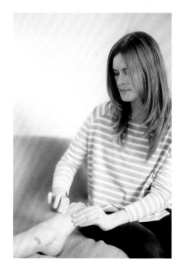

VITAMIN PILLS
& OTHER SUPPLEMENTS

I have never really taken vitamin pills regularly or consistently. I felt that with a good diet that included juices, smoothies, lots of dark vegetables, garlic, olive oil, lemon, ginger, chilli and herbs I would be ticking all the boxes on the recommended guidelines. Plus, by constantly reminding myself to keep my body alkalised I felt I should be in good shape. In fact, when I had a blood test recently I had no deficiency in anything apart from omega 3s, which is probably because I do not eat meat or fish, even though I make up for this by ensuring I get plenty of protein from non-animal sources such as tofu, lentils, tempeh, beans and pulses. Even sticking to a good diet, though, it's hard to be completely sure that we have all the vitamins and minerals we need for full health so I have listed the supplements I would advise you to keep in your fridge: vitamin C, vitamin D, magnesium, probiotics and omega 3 and 6.

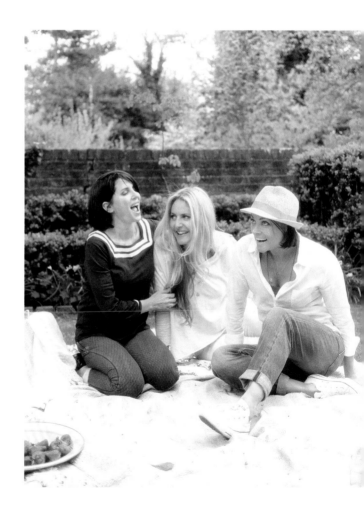

VITAMINS

to be or not to be?

Vitamin C

Vitamin C, also called ascorbic acid, is a water-soluble nutrient found in some foods. In the body it acts as an antioxidant, protecting cells from the damage caused by free radicals. Free radicals are compounds formed when our bodies convert food we consume into energy. We are also exposed to free radicals every day by things such as cigarette smoke, air pollution and ultra violet light from the sun.

Our bodies need Vitamin C to make collagen, a protein that is required to help wounds heal. It also helps the immune system to work properly and protects the body from disease. Vitamin C can also improve your body's ability to absorb iron.

Vitamin D

Vitamin D is important for growth, good health and strong bones. The main reason for taking vitamin D is to aid the absorption of calcium and phosphorus as they are what keep our bones strong.

Most of our vitamin D comes from exposure to sunlight during the summer months – the vitamin is made by our body in reaction to the sunlight. During winter months, people living in temperate climates like the UK can lack vitamin D because they don't get enough sunlight to the skin. We mustn't get confused with sunbathing for our dose of vitamin D: too much exposure to the sun can cause sunburn, premature ageing of the skin and lead to skin cancer. So make sure your exposure to the sun is for just 10–15 minutes. The best time of day for absorbing vitamin D is between 11am and 3pm.

In winter months when sun exposure is hard to get, I advise you to take a supplement. Ask in your health store which one they recommend.

Foods rich in vitamin C:
Broccoli, Brussels sprouts, Cauliflower, Kale, Lemon Juice, Oranges, Papaya, Parsley, Red and Green Peppers, Strawberries, Tomatoes

Foods rich in vitamin D:
Eggs, Mackerel, Sardines

Foods rich in magnesium:
Avocado, Fish, Garlic, Green Leafy Vegetables, Nuts (especially almonds), Parsley, Whole Grains such as Brown Rice, Buckwheat, Millet, Barley

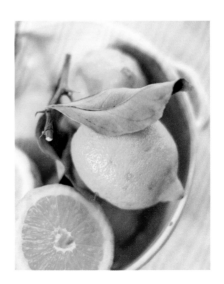

Magnesium

Magnesium is essential to the maintenance of healthy bones and teeth because it is needed for the release of calcitonin, the hormone that encourages calcium to be deposited into the bones. Magnesium offers lots of other health benefits, which include transmission of nerve impulses, body temperature regulation, detoxification, and energy production. It can also help with migraines, insomnia, and depression. Taking magnesium supplements has been found to help with panic attacks, stress, anxiety and agitations. Magnesium is such an important mineral that we need to make sure that we get our daily dose. Sixty per cent of magnesium in the body is within our bones and 26 per cent is in our muscles, the remainder being soft tissue and body fluids. Apart from taking supplements to ensure you are getting enough, I have found that soaking in a magnesium salt bath works wonders. Better You (www.betteryou. uk.com) sell a great range of magnesium products. Magnesium is absorbed through the skin while you bathe and this is a great way to speed up recovery after a workout. The magnesium helps to produce serotonin, a mood-elevating chemical within the brain that creates a feeling of calm. Magnesium can also reduce irritability by lowering the effects of adrenaline. It can create a relaxed feeling, improve sleep and concentration, and help muscles and nerves to function properly.

Try to limit your intake of coffee, salt, sugar and alcohol as they increase the excretion of magnesium through urine, thus depleting the magnesium stored in your body.

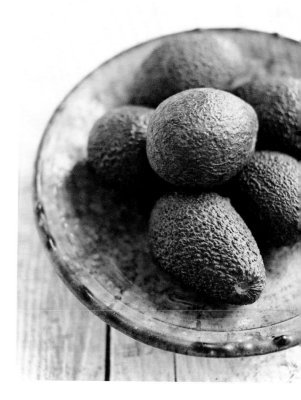

PH LEVELS

I think it is very important to look at your acid and alkaline imbalance and you can do this by buying some pH strips and following the instructions. (These strips, which can be ordered online, will give you a clear indication of where your body is on the acid and alkaline scale and how it changes throughout the day.) An imbalance in your pH can cause minor ailments and more serious ones can develop later if not corrected. Among these are cardiovascular damage, poor immune system, joint pains, osteoporosis, hormone concerns and premature ageing.

There are some very simple steps you can take to balance your pH levels and moderate them so you are keeping your body mainly alkalised. Our bodies have to keep the pH of our blood, cells and other fluid at just slightly alkaline (pH 7.365). What happens when we eat a diet high in acidic foods such as fizzy drinks, chocolate, crisps, etc. is that the body has to draw upon its own store of alkaline buffers to neutralise the acid-forming effects of our diet. As an example, if we eat a very acidic diet then our bodies need more calcium from the body, which can lead to osteoporosis. By eating foods that are alkaline we don't have to draw on supplies within our bodies and we will be much healthier.

One of the things you can do to counter too much acid in the body is to drink lots of water. I always drink hot water and lemon on waking.

Alkaline foods and drinks:
Asparagus, Broccoli, Garlic, Grapefruit, Herbal tea, Lemon, Lemon water, Lime, Mango, Olive Oil, Onion, Papaya, Parsley, Raw Spinach, Vegetable Juices, Watermelon

Foods and drinks that should definitely be avoided:
Beef, Beer, Chocolate, Cheese, Coffee, Ice Cream, Pastries, Pasta, Pork, Shellfish, Soft Drinks, Sugar (white or brown), Wheat, White flour, White rice

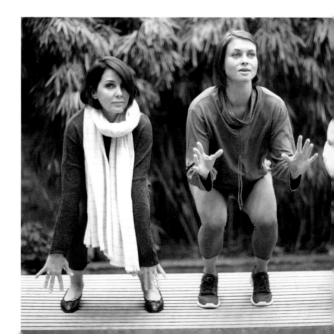

PROBIOTICS
& OMEGAS

Probiotics

Probiotics are microorganisms such as bacteria or yeasts that are believed to improve health. The digestive system is home to more than 500 different types of bacteria or microflora which help to keep our intestines healthy, assist in digestion and maintain a strong immune system. If we take a course of antibiotics or we get an infection in the body, the balance of friendly bacteria in our gut can become disturbed. Taking probiotics can improve the function of the intestines and may also help fight bacteria that cause diarrhoea.

Natural yogurt contains probiotics or you can buy supplements from your local health store. I really strongly advise you take these to keep your digestion healthy and boost your immune system.

Omegas 3 & 6

Omegas are essential for brain function, vision, learning ability, mood and co-ordination. Having the correct level of omegas may prevent and control a number of inflammatory conditions such as heart disease, arthritis, and immune dysfunction (e.g. asthma and eczema)

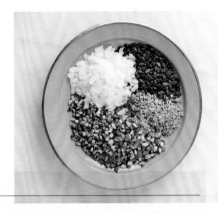

There are good levels of omega 3s in:
Flax, Hemp, Pumpkin, Walnut

Omega 6s occur in:
Safflower, Sesame, Sunflower, Sweetcorn

I take a vegetarian supplement called blue algae, but you could also take fish oil to ensure you get your omegas. Ask in a health store which one they recommend.

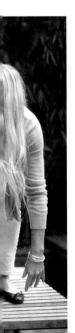

WELL WOMAN

It is very important to look after every aspect of yourself, from your diet to your body, mind and soul! I have done as much self-care as I can, but I have also had a lot of help from teachers, natural healers and conventional doctors.

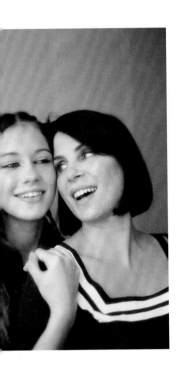

Health checks

I have always been very up front about having health checks, getting my bloods done, pelvic checks, keeping up to date and familiar with my breast care, dental visits and observing the changes in my skin, such as sun damage and moles. By implementing these medical checks regularly you stay on top of your health and wellness so if any problems do arise you can immediately take action. As a young woman I had many scares and problems relating to the health of my breasts and pelvic area. This led me to have thorough and regular screening: scans, mammograms, cervix and uterus care and regular smears to detect pre-cancerous cells, among other things. These checks have probably helped save my life, so that correct treatment could be carried out without delay.

I was lucky enough to be under the care of the medical pioneer Yehudi Gordon, who was consultant gynaecologist at Viveka, a women's health care practice in north London that, sadly, is no longer there. Yehudi has advised and acted as consultant for me for 25 years from early womanhood to being a mature woman four kids later.

He has taught me a great deal both spiritually and physically and I owe an awful lot to him. So if there's any advice that you should take from me, it is to make sure you keep up to date with all your medical checks.

From menstruation to menopause, every stage in a woman's life can be delicate, sensitive and different. Hormones can control so much of our lives both emotionally and physically and so to get a better understanding of this I recommend you read up in detail more about these topics. I highly recommend *The Good Birth Companion* by Yehudi Gordon & Nicole Croft, *Birth and Beyond* by Yehudi Gordon and *The Natural Health Bible for Women* by Dr Marilyn Glenville.

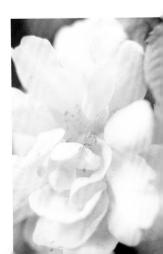

Pelvic checks

Women between the ages of 25 and 64 years should have an annual smear test (cervical screening/pelvic check). Cervical screening is used to check the cells in the cervix (neck of the womb) for any abnormalities that could lead to cancer. It is important to also look out for unusual symptoms. If you have any of the following, it is best to speak to a doctor straight away: painful intercourse, an odd-smelling discharge, persistent pelvic pain or unexpected bleeding, unusual dryness or an increased amount of discharge.

Breast checks

Check your own breasts at home every month. Visit the NHS website, which gives a great explanation of how to do this. It is important to check your breasts every month and if anything feels worrying, see your doctor. It is better to be safe and if breast cancer is diagnosed, the sooner it is treated the better chance of success.

You need to see a doctor straight away if you notice any of the following: a change in size and shape of your breast, especially if you notice this when you move your arm or lift your breast, a rash around your nipple, a red moist area on your nipple that won't heal easily, discharge from your nipple that is not milky, bleeding from your nipple, any pain or discomfort in your breasts or arm pit that won't go away, a new lump on one breast that is not on the same place as the opposite breast, or if your skin looks or feels different, for example dimpling or puckering.

Blood tests

There are a number of blood tests that can be done to assess your general health, and to check how well organs such as the liver and kidneys are functioning. Blood tests just take a few minutes and can be done by a nurse at your GP's surgery or at a hospital. It is a good idea to have them done every year, especially as you get older.

Urine tests

They are very useful for detecting problems with the kidneys and urinary tract system, diabetes and bladder cancer. If you notice any blood in your urine, tell your GP straight away.

Sexual health

The best way to keep yourself safe from infections or passing any on is by using a condom. Get tested for sexually transmitted diseases before you start any new relationship. At an STI clinic they can test for HIV, chlamydia, herpes, syphilis and gonorrhoea.

Diabetes

If there is a history of diabetes in your family or your BMI is greater than 25, you should get your haemoglobin A1c checked. The Haemoglobin A1c Test gives you an average blood sugar level over the last three months rather than just at one point in time.

Blood pressure

It is really important to get this checked regularly because high blood pressure can put a strain on your arteries and heart, which means you will be more likely to suffer a stroke, heart attack or kidney disease. Get your blood pressure checked at least once a year. If it has been abnormally high or low then you need to check it more frequently.

Cholesterol check

Cholesterol is a fat that is carried around in our bodies and exists in all our cell membranes. Eighty per cent of cholesterol is produced by the liver and 20 per cent derives directly from the food we eat. If your cholesterol is too high, it can block the arteries and increase your risk of heart disease and strokes. Make sure you get tested every 3–5 years.

Eye tests

Regular eye tests are very important because your eyes don't usually hurt if something is wrong. Optometrists can detect the early signs of certain eye conditions before you are even aware of symptoms. You might need glasses for the first time or you may need a different prescription for the glasses you already have. They can also pick up on early signs of diabetes, glaucoma and macular degeneration. So do have your eyes tested every two years or more frequently if it has been advised by your doctor.

Dentist

Brush your teeth with fluoride toothpaste twice a day. Floss your teeth daily and remember that smoking, sugary drinks and sugary food will affect the health of your teeth and gums. So the healthier you are, the longer your teeth will last. Go for a check-up once a year but if you are prone to tooth decay then it is suggested to visit every 6 months.

Skin checks and moles

Look for changes in your skin and moles monthly and get a yearly skin check from your doctor. If you notice any changes to your moles – in colour, size, if they are itchy, bleeding or they have an irregular shape – then you must see your doctor straight away.

Pregnancy, babies and being a mummy

Pregnancy can be a wonderful thing in a woman's life, a time full of excitement and wonderment. I experienced it four times and all my pregnancies were completely different. I suffered from hyperemesis, a complication that causes vomiting, nausea and dehydration. I was hospitalised and put on a hydration drip until my body had recuperated and was rested. Also three out of my four babies were born at 32/33 weeks, which meant their first few hours or days were spent in an incubator. So, even though having my children is the most wonderful thing I have done in my life, I know pregnancy and childbirth can also be complicated and stressful.

I took a natural approach to my pregnancies and to the births but in no way would I judge the different choices women make: every woman is different, as is every pregnancy. What worked for me, though, was sticking to yoga, reflexology, positive thinking and visualisation as well as meditation, all of which are discussed in this book. These different therapies helped me with my pregnancies and the actual labour (I opted for water-births). I tried to eat healthily and stick to my normal diet as much as possible, never giving myself a hard time if I craved only sweets and jelly babies because when you are struggling with morning sickness you have to, to some extent, follow your cravings.

Beautiful baby

Motherhood is like nothing else, the love you feel is beyond your expectations and when you see your beautiful innocent child suddenly your life makes sense. The first few nights when I took my baby home and got to know this new human being were, to me, what dreams are made of. Of course motherhood is tiring and stressful, as you have to learn on your feet how to parent your child all the way from being a defenceless little baby to adulthood – mostly without any training. So a lot of it must be instinctive to you and again a very personal thing.

Being a mummy

When my children were born I chose that they slept in bed with me. I also chose not to let them cry themselves to sleep, and I never ignored them when they were crying and wanted something. Yes, it did mean parenting was a lot harder as I had to attend to their every need and be very hands on. But as with any stage in life, you just get on with it and face problems head on. There are highs and lows and I experienced both, including lows when I suffered from severe postnatal depression and was even hospitalised on some occasions. It was over eleven years ago when I suffered from postnatal depression and at that time there were quite a few stigmas attached to the condition. For many people it was as if you were behaving like a moaning minnie who should be grateful and not complain that you had a beautiful baby in your arms. The simplest way I can describe it is to say that there is no rationale behind it, it hits you hard and you may experience some of the darkest and scariest days of your life, feeling cut off, lonely and possibly unsupported. If you have any concerns that you may have postnatal depression please see your doctor immediately and be reassured there is treatment that will make you feel better. In time, the feelings you have will pass and you will be able to get on with your life.

Motherhood has many different phases, from the cooing baby, the energetic toddler, the questioning and curious infant, to the rebellious and sometimes worrying teenager. You have to evolve with them and try your best to give them unconditional love. I have in no way been the perfect mother and have made many mistakes as we all have. But I have loved my children constantly and tried not to judge and expect unrealistic things from them. To me, being a mother involves teaching my children about the good things in life, being compassionate, generous and forgiving but also accepting that, at the end of the day, they have to find their own way and learn by their own mistakes

– especially in their teenage years when they find you highly embarrassing and do not listen to a word you say. Above all, I try to stress to my children to have no judgement and to be loyal and loving to themselves.

Family matters and therapy

What is a normal family? What family has a completely normal set up these days? It is sad but true, what family has not suffered some tragedy, misfortune or scandal? Life is complicated, painful and, without sounding too much like a hippy, we are on a journey, experiencing life on life's terms and learning lessons every day.

The dynamics of each family are different and can be constantly evolving. Sometimes we can get into unhealthy patterns so it can be helpful to get some extra help from someone who is experienced, like a therapist. Whether you are facing things on your own or with a partner or even the whole family, problems can be shifted, aired and then hopefully remedied.

I have used therapy during various points in my life – when I lost my father, when I was going through a painful break up and when I had postnatal depression. Looking back, I can say now that with the work I put into my therapy, my whole life seems less complicated and a whole lot better.

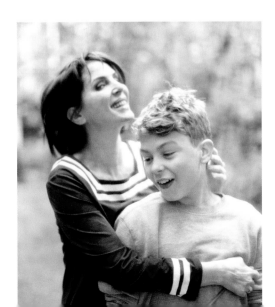

Joint custody and step-parenting

Separation, divorce, joint custody of children plus step-parenting is becoming more and more a part of the modern family. Very few separations are easy and they bring turmoil, change and sometimes a lot of pain. It is a highly transitional period and requires a long time for everyone to adjust. Both adults and children have a lot of changes to deal with; everything becomes a very different world. There can be a lot of tears and fights but also the possibility of new and fresh beginnings, which in the long run will make everyone happier.

Then divorce may come, which can be incredibly stressful and destructive. Sometimes it becomes a mini personal war in which no one is the winner apart from the lawyers. Try your hardest to resist petty arguments and mind games and if you see yourself becoming bitter and negative, surround yourself with white light as well as the person you are having problems with. This will create better vibes between you and create a more karmic situation. It can be quite challenging if you have to separate and divorce, dividing your time and splitting up your family. At first your family doesn't feel like your family. It is such a loss and time of grieving when you see your child/children less because it is your ex's turn. I had to throw myself into lots of different things such as hobbies and work hard at keeping an exciting social life including meeting new people. I took up rock-climbing, trapeze, script writing and started new businesses, which was all quite exhausting but also liberating.

Another area we are not prepared for is that of being a step-parent. With the little experience I have had, you should be open, generous, kind, delicate and never push. Children will always pick up on it if an adult is pushing too hard and not being genuine. So make sure you are not demanding and that you are instinctive and not trying to buy their affection through presents.

No judgement

Judgement can be a very destructive trait. Either to judge yourself or to judge others will only give you inner angst and conflict. So when you notice yourself being critical or having judgemental thoughts about others, try to correct yourself: what works for me is if I tell myself to mind my own business – I immediately stop. Or, if I am beating myself up and judging myself, I think 'would I be so hard on someone I love so much, like my daughter?' I must love myself as much as one of my loved ones and stop having negative thoughts about myself as that too will only create negative situations.

Positivity

Always try and make every situation as positive as possible. Be as positive as you can and try to have positive thoughts. By doing this your life will be more contented and peaceful.

Conclusion

There is a certain love and care that we should all give ourselves daily. There are many traps we can all fall into but there is a way to make things easier, more fun, so you can live a life of contentment. We all try to practise what we preach but if for some reason things become a little unmanageable and we develop some bad habits, we have to draw a line under it and start again! I hope our book has given some insight into healthy food, exercise and life in general.

Protect your mind, body and soul and love thy self and neighbour.

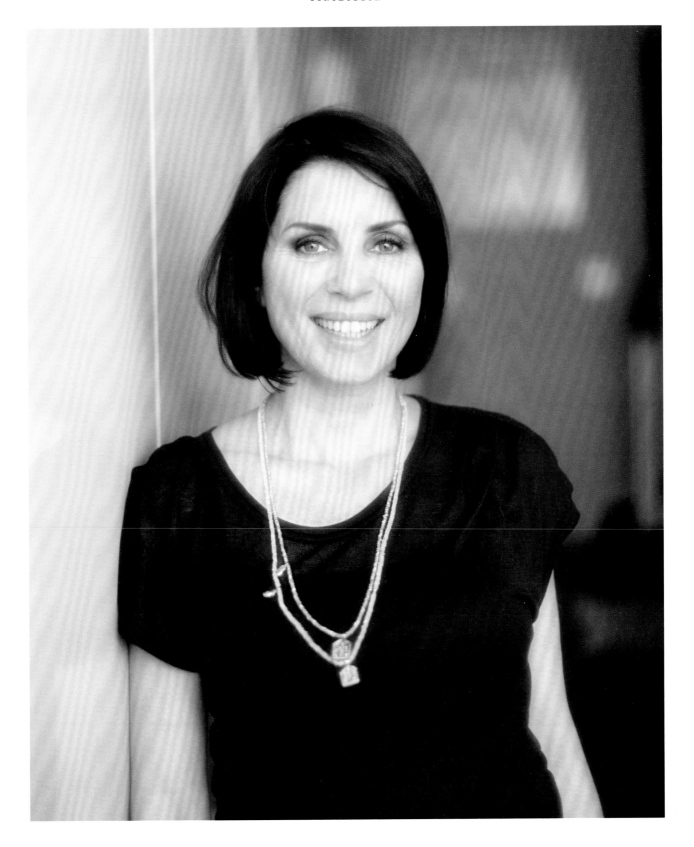

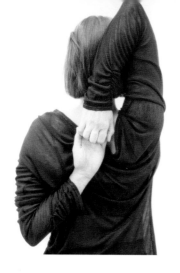

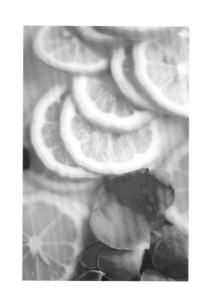

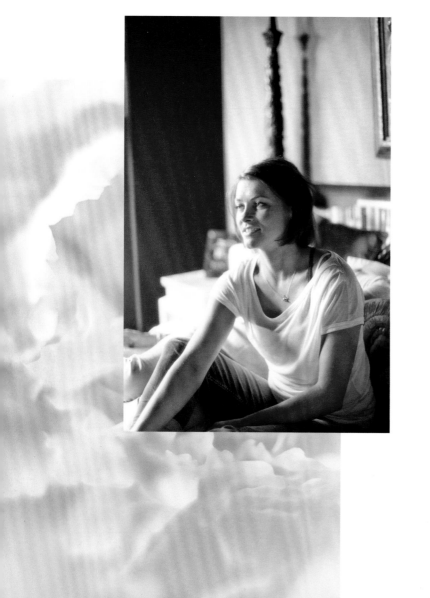

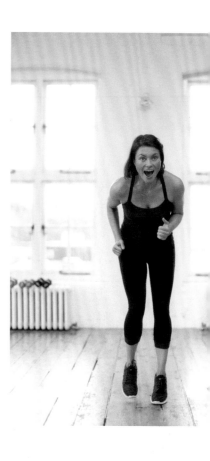

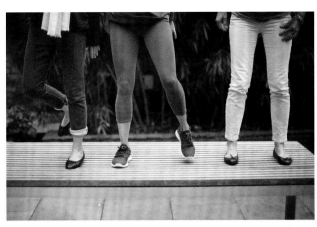

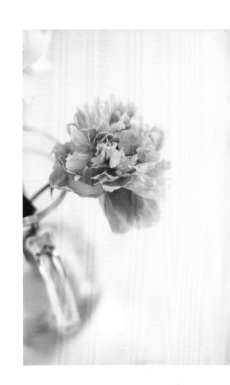

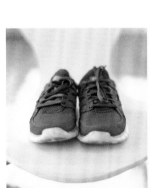

FIT-WOMAN

Holly

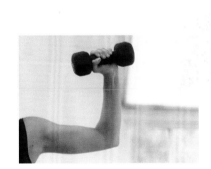

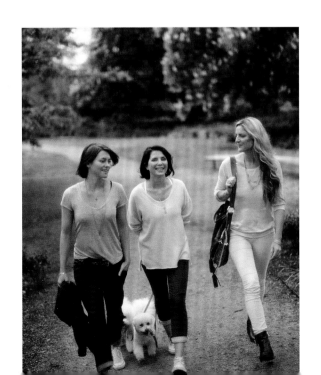

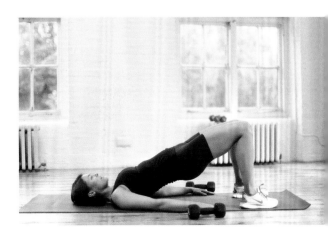

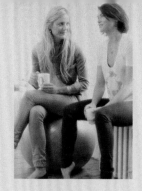

I have spent many years as a personal trainer and lifestyle coach to hundreds of people. Some are ordinary women and men wanting to be fitter, some are postnatal women who want to feel body-confident again, some are actors preparing for film roles, and some are people who want to change their bad habits. I've individually tailored each programme, but the fundamental principle is the same: discover a healthy lifestyle, and fall in love with exercise.

I'm not talking quick fixes here, there is no secret powder or magic smoothie. I'm talking about long-lasting, maintainable changes that come from a holistic reboot of bad habits.

By sharing my passion and knowledge of fitness and nutrition, I have given my clients the confidence they need to pursue a healthy and active lifestyle. Small changes lead to big differences in terms of happiness, confidence and weight loss. Learn better habits, and break the bad ones. Most importantly, I teach my clients how to make it all last.

The fundamental principle is the same: discover a healthy lifestyle, and fall in love with exercise.

I was brought up vegetarian and from the age of six I lived in the countryside. We had a massive vegetable garden, so I was introduced to a delicious variety of fresh, seasonal vegetables and had hands-on experience of planting and picking home-grown produce. Watching your food grow from seed and knowing where it has come from helps you appreciate it. I have wonderful memories of podding fresh peas in the summer and digging up the first of the new potatoes, washing off the dirt, watching them boil and then popping those sweet, delicious, buttery spuds into my mouth. Heaven.

But 'vegetarian' does not equal 'healthy' and being vegetarian does not automatically imply you follow a varied and healthy diet. When I left home for London, convenience drove my diet and things changed. I replaced all the fresh seasonal vegetables with frozen potato waffles, ready-made vegetable pies and easy pasta dishes. It was a slippery slope, my taste began to gravitate to sweet and sugary foods. As a young actress, I found myself out socialising an awful lot and began to smoke and drink too much.

I suffered from colds and coughs all the time and began to feel sluggish, bloated and low in energy. Eating left me with a horrible stuffed feeling. At 25 I knew I was out of balance.

I was active, yet far from healthy, and was not happy. I started trying different diets, the cabbage soup diet being particularly dissatisfying. I would feel good for a week or so but couldn't sustain the discipline of such extreme diets so would revert back to bingeing on chocolate (I have always had a sweet tooth) and fall back into my unhealthy habits. This cycle needed to change.

I began reading many healthy eating books. I found them interesting and inspiring and, the more I learnt, the more things began to fall into place. It didn't

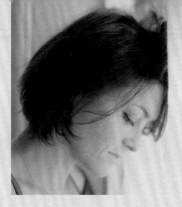

happen overnight. Bad habits often tend to become ingrained much faster than good ones. But slowly I started to make changes – lasting changes. I learned about raw food, food combining, juice fasting, GI (glycaemic index) and toxic foods. I began cookery and nutrition courses, which is when I realised I wanted to become a personal trainer. Something very profound happened. In correcting my own bad habits I realised the joy and deep satisfaction it can provide, and I needed to share it.

I finally made the connection between foods with no nutritional value and the fact that I was feeling sluggish and getting ill. After countless hours and years of work, the two key things that helped me find the balance I was missing were: having the knowledge to know what to eat and how to work out; and understanding how to use it to make it part of my everyday routine. The more I read and learned about what I was eating and drinking and the long-term effect it was having on my body and overall health, the less I wanted to pollute myself. Today, I make the choice to eat healthy food because it makes me feel good from the inside out. When I eat a nutritious, freshly cooked meal, I feel happy. It's that simple. Drinking hot water with fresh lemon in the morning means I start the day feeling energised. I don't give in to guilt when I occasionally eat dark chocolate or have a glass of wine because overall I know my diet is healthy and balanced.

I have always been active. As a child I climbed trees, ran through fields and jumped on my trampoline in the garden. When I moved to London at 17, I joined a gym and started practising yoga (my sister Sadie took me to my first class). In the spirit of balance I sought a high-energy alternative to yoga and soon became hooked on kickboxing. Motivation to exercise has always been easy for me, and just like jumping on my trampoline,

it's because I have chosen things I love to do. I have never considered staying fit to be a chore. When you see kids constantly moving, jumping, skipping, running – they are doing it because it's fun, they're loving every moment of it.

If I don't like a particular form of exercise, I won't do it – there's another one that I do like. Trying new teachers, new places to train and new people to train with is all part of the process. I won't give up if things are a bit hard or challenging, I like to push myself and you soon know if what you are doing works for you.

I used to think that life happened in the future; I raced forward, always planning ahead and never truly being present in the moment. Get-up-and-go is easy for me but slowing myself down has been more challenging – and not just physically. It has been just as important for me to become aware of my mind and inner self. Yoga has really helped me achieve this balance. I started practising yoga to become fitter, but now I use it to slow myself down and be present in the moment. Mindfulness and meditation courses have also helped to ground me. I love reading books that bring me back to the present and help me live my life more in the moment. It's a constant process of learning and growing.

Love Holly xxx

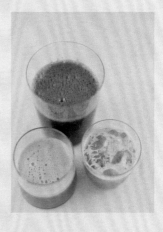

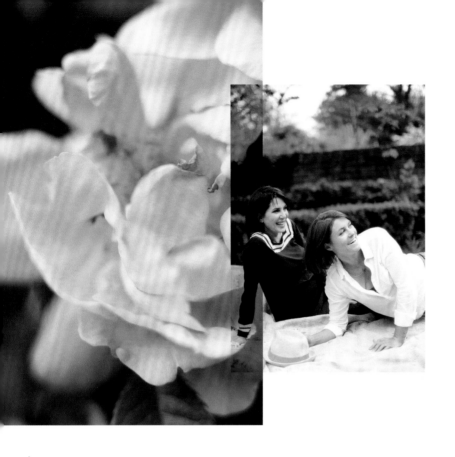
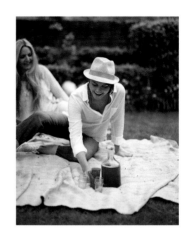
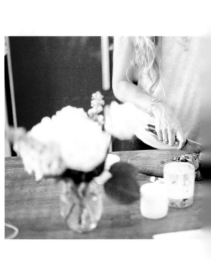
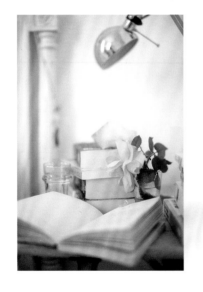
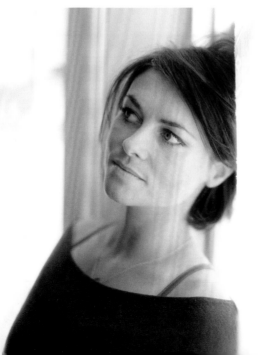

MINDSET

I now know what has enabled me to become healthy, both physically and mentally, emotionally balanced, stress-free and content. In summary it is about:

- **Being active**
- **Enjoying a daily variety of fresh vegetables**
- **Limiting my intake of sugar, wheat and alcohol**
- **Avoiding processed foods and always reading food labels**
- **Having 'me' time**
- **Not taking life too seriously and having fun**
- **Trying new things to keep me sharp, excited and inspired**
- **Being with positive, like-minded people who nurture a zest for life**

You do have a choice, you can learn about which are the best foods for your health and for weight loss – Amber's delicious recipes will get you on track. You can also find the exercise you find enjoyable and see how you can become strong, lean and toned. Don't underestimate the importance of having time for yourself, time to rest, relax and just be.

Every one of us can wake up in the morning and say that today, right now, this second I am in control and I love the way I am. Are you ready?

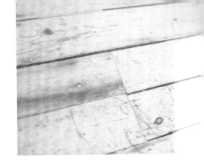

CHANGING
HABITS

It's great to embark on a healthy lifestyle and a new fitness regime, feeling excited and inspired. But it's so easy to want it all to happen instantly, the good old 'I want it now' syndrome. So you bust a gut and cram in exercise every day. By the end of the first week you are aching but still feel positive; by the end of the second week you scream 'It's taking over my life! I hate exercise!' and throw in the towel. If you haven't exercised before or been able to maintain exercise over a long period of time, then going at it hard won't be sustainable. Far better to ease into it slowly and build it up gradually, until exercising eventually becomes part of your weekly routine. It won't happen overnight.

It's time to ditch some bad habits, too. How often when you look in the mirror do you focus straight away on what you don't like about your body? If you have negative thoughts about parts of yourself they are often what your eyes are first drawn to: my thighs are too big, my arms are flabby, I hate the shape of my butt. Be positive about yourself and change the habit. Whenever you look in the mirror, make a point of focusing on a positive feature and pay yourself at least one compliment. Highlight your natural gifts, talent, and abilities and don't just rate yourself in terms of appearance.

Changing habits and creating a motivational mindset is like exercising a muscle – the more you work it, the stronger it becomes. Some of our behaviours and thoughts have been with us all of our lives, so it takes time.

Little things like associating the word 'treat' with food (quite likely rubbish, fatty, sugary food). Most of us have the connection from when we were children and our mums would give us sweets as a reward if we behaved ourselves. There are other ways to be rewarded: treat yourself to a walk in the park or indulge in reading a good book.

EXERCISING EVENTUALLY
BECOMES PART OF YOUR
WEEKLY ROUTINE. IT WON'T
HAPPEN OVERNIGHT.

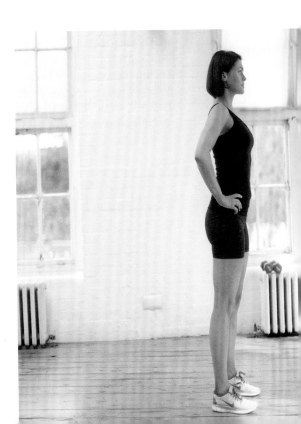

TAKE THE
PRESSURE OFF

Taking the pressure off yourself is so important. If you are told not to do something, you kind of want to do it (watch your kids, they're expert at this). As soon as you restrict your diet, all you want to do is eat. And when you tell yourself you HAVE to do a workout, you feel pressured and try to talk yourself out of it. There is no pressure. There is no stress. If you only do half a workout then please congratulate yourself, that's great! Likewise, if you manage a brisk walk around the park, amazing – it's all about moving, getting your body active. Yes, becoming fitter, stronger or leaner can seem like a long journey. So don't feel you have to go at it for hours and hours, break it up into 20-minute blasts, start off small and build up when your fitness improves. Exercising without stress or pressure attached to it makes it a choice and enjoyable.

Some training programmes put you under pressure even before you begin with dubious promises: Get a dancer's body by doing this workout. Mmmm, really? These workouts can be great fun but since the girl who is posing for the workout shots has been a dancer for the last 15 years, of course she has a dancer's body and, when you don't get a body like hers, you think you have failed. Not only is it unrealistic, frankly most of us don't have the genetic makeup to have that dancer's physique. Have your own personal goals laid out. You want to be

fit and healthy for you, because that's what makes you feel good and gives you a huge sense of achievement.

Every time you work out or go to a yoga class will be different, because you are different each day. You may not have slept well; you might be more stressed or dehydrated. Don't get angry if today is harder or isn't the same as the last time you trained. Do the best you can do today, don't focus on what you did yesterday or last week but on what you are doing right now. Because your best effort today is good enough.

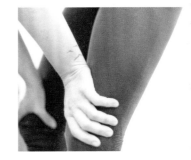

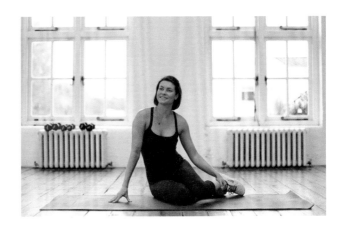

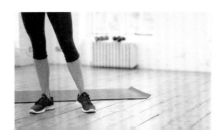

CHANGING THE VOICE
IN YOUR HEAD

We can make things into huge obstacles and we love to have a conversation with the voice in our head about it. You know the one that tells you it is OK to have a second biscuit, but then the same one that makes you feel guilty afterwards? It's a continuous chatter we have with ourselves about most things.

The voice

'I've had such a stressful day at work, I need a glass of wine tonight. I know I said I wasn't going to drink all week, but after the nightmare day I've had, I deserve it. Plus, I didn't drink last night, so that's pretty good, so I can probably have a couple.'

'I'm so tired I can't be bothered to go to the gym today. But I didn't go yesterday and I promised myself I would go today, so I'm going!... Oh, but it's pouring with rain outside, it must be a sign to stay at home. I will go tomorrow.'

WHATEVER THE MIND CAN
CONCEIVE AND BELIEVE,
IT CAN ACHIEVE.

NAPOLEON HILL.

To create a healthier lifestyle, not only do we need to change the food we eat and become more active and less stressed, but we also need to change the voice in our head to help us get there. Next time you hear the voice, don't let it talk you out of doing something positive. Try and change it to encourage and motivate you: 'I can make time', 'I feel so energised after a workout', 'It's a bit cold outside today, but I will soon warm up.'

Finding what excites you will really help to keep the voices at bay. Discover which exercises or activities you're naturally good at and do them – swimming, jogging with friends, jogging on your own, dancing, yoga, a martial art or exercise class, Pilates or playing football with your kids. Keep trying new things until you find the right ones, and accept you may need to find a great teacher who inspires you or the perfect class that fits into your schedule.

We all have days when it's harder to motivate ourselves but those sessions can turn out to be more rewarding as you know you have made the extra effort.

I still have days when my little voice raises its ugly head and I don't fancy going for a run. So I have a chat with myself (now I sound slightly crazy) to remind myself how good it makes me feel, the huge sense of achievement I get afterwards, the fresh air on my face, the freedom it gives me. The positives always outweigh the negatives. I change the voice from 'Don't bother today, you deserve a rest' to 'If I only run for 10 minutes today then that's great' and as soon as my feet hit the pavement, I know I've made the right choice and usually that 10 minutes turns into an hour.

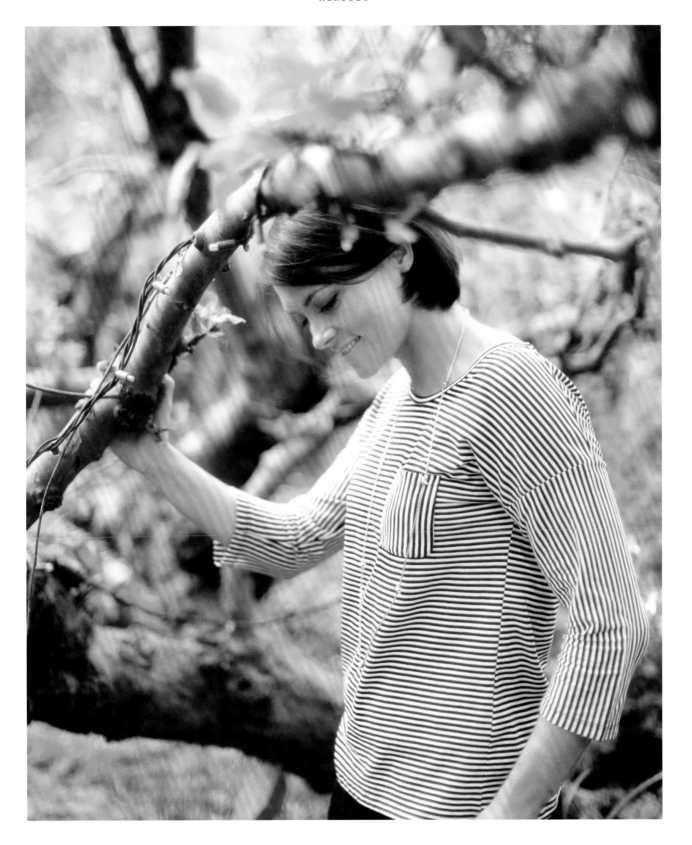

POSITIVE
THOUGHTS

In the words of Buddha, 'we are what we think'. Having a positive outlook on life brings many health benefits, from reducing stress to enhancing relationships. Positive thinking has an impact on overall well-being. In our daily lives we can encounter negativity – fear, worry, dispute, jealousy, gossip, judgement – and too often it's easy to get caught up in it and then negative thoughts become a habit. Instead, try to see the glass as half full. Set your goal and visualise yourself achieving it, be it running that race or fitting into that LBD. Having a positive attitude about exercise will boost your motivation and help you achieve your goals more easily.

Avoid negative thoughts
Don't put yourself down. Work on making your mind and body strong, remember it's you inside who says you can't do something, so challenge those negative thoughts and turn them into positives. Read inspiring, uplifting quotes. Find one that touches you and make it your mantra.

Be in the present
Focus your thoughts on the right now and be mindful of what is going on around you.

Be thankful
Focus every night on the things for which you are grateful and highlight all the good things in your life.

Learn to say no
By not over-committing to things, you're less likely to let people down or feel you have failed.

Surround yourself with other positive people
They will support and energise you. Being positive is contagious, in the same way as being negative is, and I know which people I'd choose to be around.

Smile
It's simple but it works.

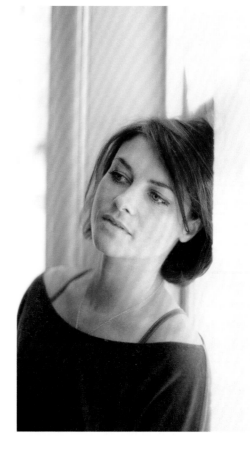

IF IT'S IMPORTANT TO YOU,
YOU WILL FIND A WAY. IF NOT,
YOU WILL FIND AN EXCUSE.

NO EXCUSES!

There are many excuses that crop up when it comes to exercising but there are always solutions, too. Do you recognise any of these excuses?

'I don't have enough time'
Even if it's a 10-minute blast we all can find time in our day for that – every minute helps. That's 70 minutes a week, 3,640 minutes a year. And that's a lot of extra calories burnt as well as a lot of endorphins – the happy hormones – released! Remember this is YOUR health and happiness you're investing in.

'I can't afford it'
You don't have to be a member of an expensive gym or invest in top of-the-range gym equipment. All you need is your body (OK, a pair of trainers and a sports bra would be great, too).

'I'm not fit enough'
That's in your head; you are fit enough. Everyone began somewhere. Start at a level that works for you and build on it.

'It's too hard'
Begin with some gentle exercise and, as your fitness improves, so too will your confidence and your ability to push yourself harder.

'I don't enjoy it'
Maybe you are doing the wrong activity: it's time to try something new.

'No clean gym kit'
Always be prepared. Double up on your kit so you always have one clean set; get it ready the night before so you're not rushing around in the morning.

'I've got a baby so I can't make it to the gym'
Home workouts and DVDs are a great way to get back into shape post-baby. If that's not for you, then you can power walk/jog pushing the buggy through the park. Find another mum who also wants to get back into shape and do babysitting swaps.

'I'm just too tired'
Exercise is proven to increase your energy levels. Change the thought of 'I'm too tired' into 'this is really going to energise and refresh me'.

'I'm injured*/I'm ill'
OK, if it's serious maybe your body needs a rest: listen to what it's telling you. Perhaps focus on something to help prevent further injury; it might be the perfect opportunity to try something new.

*If you have an injury, ache or pain, don't push through the pain – see a physio or doctor. Your body and health come first; make it a priority to get a proper diagnosis, not an excuse to stop you from working out.

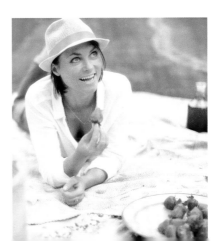

OBSTACLES

jump them all

Don't just focus on the things you are good at (we all have our favourite moves). Working on your weaker areas will help give you a strong and toned body. So when you see the exercise 'Burpee' (page 236) in front of you (most people's least favourite move) say, 'Yeah baby, bring it on!!'. Keep pushing your body, it's easy to sit back into a comfort zone. You will be surprised how much your body is capable of and how quickly you will improve. Your workouts should never be easy. In fact, when they start to feel easier it's time to make your workout more challenging. You can do this in many ways, by adding more weight, more time or more reps. Feel the burn and fall in love with it.

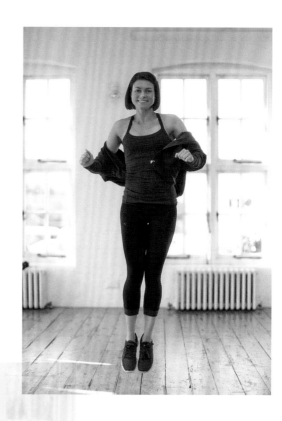

Enter a race

Nothing is more motivating than having an event on the horizon and skipping sessions becomes a lot less tempting when you've got a date set in the diary. Raise money for your favourite charity as well. That way, everyone's a winner!

Reward yourself

When you've stuck to your training plan or reached a goal, congratulate yourself. Treat yourself to a new piece of gym kit, a massage, or make time for that really relaxing candle-lit bubble bath.

Visualise achieving your goal

Feel all the emotions associated with the achievement. Really focus on the details to make this experience as real as possible.

Make a date with yourself

Commit to your weekly workouts by having them in the diary, they are just as important as any meeting.

Train with a friend

Planning to do a workout with a friend is great motivation, you are less likely to skip a workout and let down your friend and you can also spur each other on. Send a text to congratulate each other on the work you have done.

THERE WILL ALWAYS BE OBSTACLES AND REASONS NOT TO EXERCISE, AND THAT'S WHY YOU SHOULD ALWAYS HAVE A PLAN B, OR EVEN A PLAN C, IN PLACE.

Prepare playlists that motivate you

If music be the food of love then... work out!! (Isn't that what Shakespeare said?) It's proven that a pumping beat makes you work harder, so find something that makes you want to get up and go!

Buy a nice gym kit

Something you feel comfortable in, and don't put off buying it until you've lost weight. Your self-confidence might be a little low already so it's not going to do it any favours by wearing an old holey pair of tracksuit bottoms and your partner's baggy T-shirt.

Do it for them

Think of someone close to you and do the workout for them. When you feel you can't go on and you are ready to give up, visualise that special person and keep on going. Run that bit further, lift that bit heavier, do one more rep. It's not just for you anymore, it's for them, too.

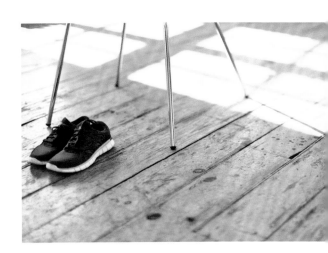

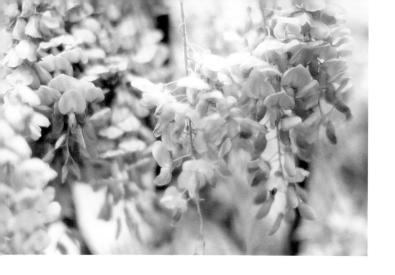

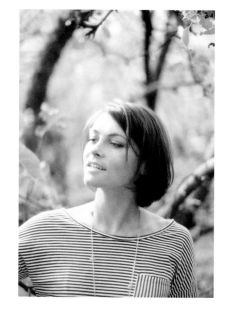

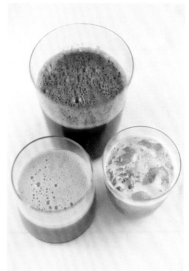

BODY

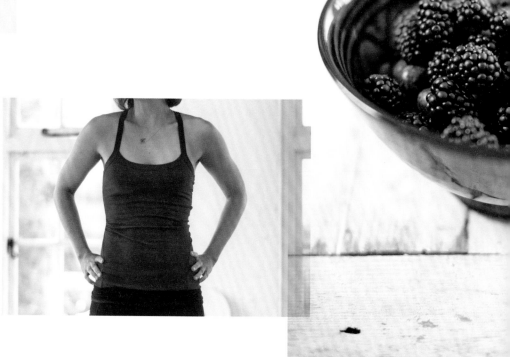

Exercise speeds up your metabolism by creating more muscle and, of course, the more intense your workout, the more calories you burn. But that does not mean exercise makes you hungrier. While a lot depends on what gender we are and our overall body composition, often we think since we've smashed our workout, we can reward ourselves with food. Mostly that's just bad habits, or your brain thinking it deserves a reward for working so hard. Studies have actually shown that the more you work out, the more you produce both appetite-suppressing proteins and hormones, so any hunger pangs might just be in your mind. Working out on an empty stomach is neither good nor bad, it's a personal choice. But what is key after exercise is making the right food choices, refuelling within an hour post-workout, and making sure it's high-quality protein to repair muscle tissue. Plus, protein makes you feel fuller longer, which is an added bonus! More important than anything is to drink plenty of water to re-hydrate your body post-workout – and water also makes you feel full. So when in doubt, grab some H_2O.

EXERCISING
& THE BENEFITS

Why do we need to exercise? The bottom line is that we need to move our bodies. That's what they are designed to do. Run, jump, push, pull, bend, reach and lift. Hundreds of years ago we didn't need to exercise – we had to be physical and active to survive. Lifts, escalators and especially cars and computers all contribute to moving less. Our bodies are wonderful machines. To function properly they need to be kept mobile, active and strong.

Staying fit isn't so easy now that practically everything is done for us. Even day-to-day chores like food shopping can all be done with a click. To top it off, there's the huge choice of food we always have available at our fingertips and the added convenience of takeaways, restaurants, cafés and ready meals. And, if we aren't preparing food ourselves, how do we really know what's in it? Not a great combo for staying fit and healthy. We need to remind ourselves why we need to be active, realise that it's not a chore but what our bodies require to thrive.

For many, weight loss is the main motivator to get in shape. But shifting the kilos is not just about trying to squeeze into your skinny jeans. The main reason for staying fit is to live a healthy life with greater confidence and self-esteem. And to be able to carry on with day-to-day activities such as running around with the kids, cleaning the house, carrying the heavy food shop, even tying our shoelaces when we are 80, feeling body-confident, living without back problems, I could go on and on…

LACK OF ACTIVITY DESTROYS THE GOOD CONDITION OF EVERY HUMAN BEING, WHILE MOVEMENT AND METHODICAL PHYSICAL EXERCISE SAVE IT AND PRESERVE IT.

PLATO

Exercise makes you feel good by releasing endorphins, the happy hormones, into your body. Just 15 minutes of exercise can improve your mood.

Exercise keeps your bones healthy – especially weight-bearing exercise, as it increases bone density, which counteracts osteoporosis.

Regular aerobic exercise lowers your blood pressure, which in turn reduces your risk of developing heart disease. Get the blood pumping and the heart racing!

Exercise speeds up your metabolism by creating more muscle. It burns body fat and calories, which will help maintain healthy weight loss. The more intense the workout the more calories you burn. So smash it!

Exercise improves your sex life – fitter people have better sex.

Exercise gives you energy. Being active or hitting the gym is invigorating – it's the best medicine for when you're feeling sluggish.

Exercise results in smoother, more radiant, younger-looking skin because it helps pump more blood all over your body, delivering reparative nutrients to your skin's surface. It also increases collagen production making your skin appear more youthful. Yes please!

Exercise reduces stress, tension, anxiety and boredom. It lowers the levels of cortisol, the stress hormone, in the body. Ever tried boxing? It's a super stress release.

Exercise increases the amount of blood and oxygen pumped to your brain, keeping it sharp and more

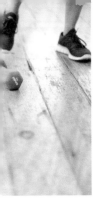

focused. Regular exercise can reduce the risk of dementia. Next time you feel mentally exhausted try a few jumping jacks to reboot your brain.

Exercise strengthens and stimulates the heart and lungs, making them work more efficiently. So you can run for the bus without becoming breathless and in the long-term you could prevent the onset of heart and lung disease.

Exercise keeps your muscles strong and your body flexible. Moving your joints regularly and keeping your muscles toned will help you continue with day-to-day activities as you get older. What you put in now will be rewarded later.

Exercise improves digestion. It helps the intestinal muscles break down food. It keeps you regular (that's the nicest way of putting it).

Regular exercise helps to prevent back pain by increasing your strength, endurance and improving your flexibility and posture. It makes you aware of the way you sit, stand and move.

You may have heard people talking about a runner's high. Let's change that saying to an 'exercise high'. I can promise you it does exist and it's pretty addictive. The first few workouts may be tough, you might feel sore, out of shape and tired, but suddenly you feel the rush – you feel strong, alive, your heart's pumping, and you feel a massive sense of achievement. When you commit to exercise your body responds quickly and you will see huge changes in your overall body shape, your sense of well-being and confidence, and your fitness in a short space of time. Chase the buzz and feel the high.

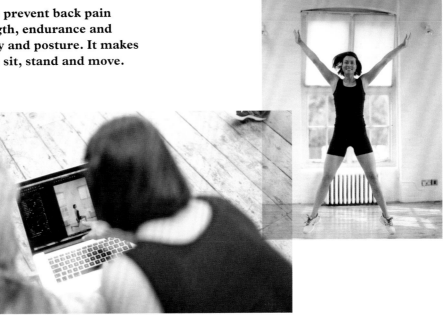

BREATHING *while* EXERCISING

Breath is life. But we take breathing for granted as we do it every second of every day without thinking about it. It's an automatic response. Breathing is the only way our blood and organs are supplied with vital oxygen. It's also one of the ways our bodies eliminate toxins and waste products. Ensuring you breathe correctly when you exercise will improve your workouts no end. When you think about it, each breath provides your muscles with fresh oxygen. Sometimes we focus so much on what we are doing we tend to hold our breath and that means our muscles are denied oxygen and everything becomes so much harder. Try to learn how to breathe for these various workouts:

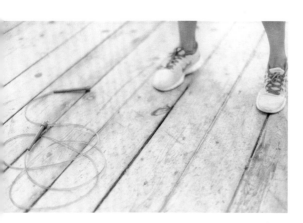

Strength training

During weight or resistance training make sure you breathe out (exhale) on the effort, which is the hardest part of the exercise – usually when you are working against gravity – and inhale on the easier part. Don't worry if you get it the wrong way round; breathing in reverse is much better than not breathing at all! Likewise, when doing a push up, inhale on the way down and exhale on the way up.

Cardio (aerobic) exercise

Take deep breaths through the diaphragm and avoid shallow breathing into the chest. You want to maintain as regular a breathing pattern as possible to maximise the oxygen flow. It doesn't matter whether you breathe through your nose or mouth or a combination of the two; everyone has a different preference.

Running

It's advisable to breathe through your mouth when running as you can take in more oxygen. Try to find a rhythm for your breathing to help keep the inhale/exhale rate consistent. Inhale every two steps then exhale on the next two, or see if a 3:3 rhythm works better for you (inhale every three steps then exhale on the following three).

Stretching

Breathing properly while you stretch will help relax your body, by bringing it back to a resting state. If you don't relax it's easy to hold your breath and put stress and more tension on the body. Take long deep breaths and inhale through your nose and exhale through your mouth. On every exhale try to relax more and give in fully to the stretch.

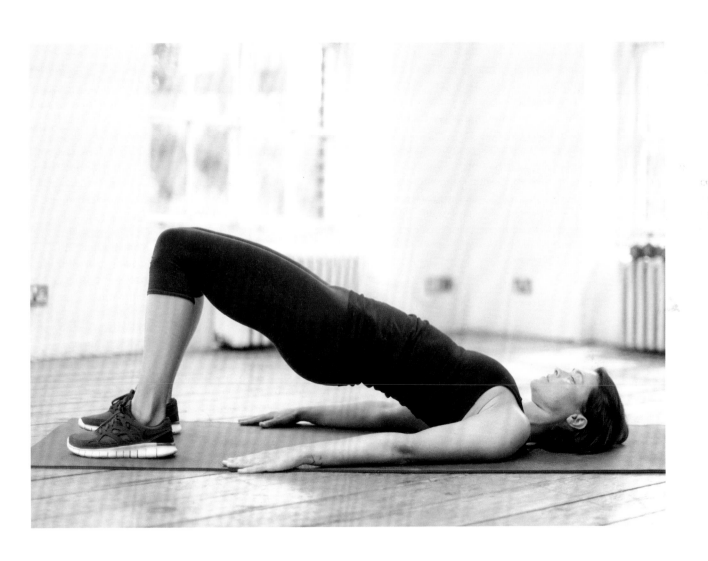

THERE IS NOTHING WORSE THAN
DOING THE SAME THING WEEK
IN, WEEK OUT.

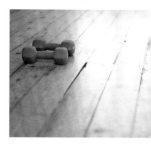

FORM, CORE
& POSTURE

Focus on the moment

Exercise offers you the perfect time to practice 'mindfulness' and be present in the moment. Whilst concentrating on your breathing, inhale and exhale to be fully present for the amazing thing you are doing for your body. Now is not the time to be working out your shopping list! This is the time to concentrate on the muscles you are working, the time to think about your toned butt, and how you are working your legs to make them lean and strong. And when it gets tough, remind yourself of the benefits of what you are doing. Tell yourself: I am becoming fitter, I am burning fat and I am making my body lean and strong.

It's all about your form

What's form, you ask? Well, it's another way of saying how you pose and position your body for each exercise. Engage your core, correct your body alignment, tighten your butt, straighten your back, that kind of thing. Form takes practice so you will want to prioritise developing it over the number of repetitions you do or how fast you can work out. Take it slowly at first. Learning good form will help you build more muscle and, more importantly, prevent injury. Always think about the muscles you are working and make sure that's where you are feeling it. Try exercising in front of a mirror. This will help increase your awareness of the way your body is moving and help to correct your form. Concentrate on all those fabulous muscles inside your body becoming strong, lean and happy!

The secret to keeping good form is working your core (your middle, stomach and back). Always keep your stomach muscles engaged and your back straight. If you feel pain in your back or joints such as your knees, chances are you are doing the exercise wrong. Check your alignment in the mirror. The only place you should feel the burn is in the muscles you are working.

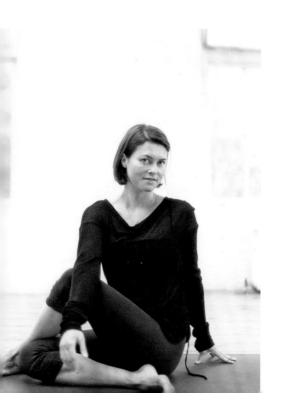

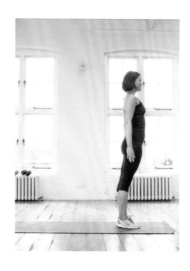

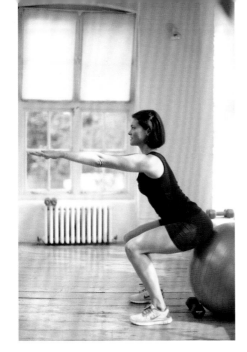

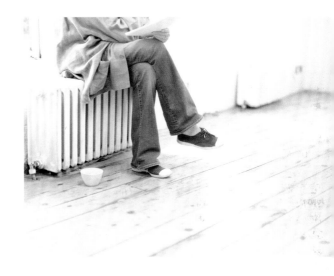

Not only is your core good for your form, it's good for your health and love life, too!
Working your core will make you strong from the inside out. We all need to work our core because it keeps the spine and pelvis stable and provides crucial support. For women, it is particularly important to strengthen the PF (pelvic floor) and TVA (transverse abdominal), especially after giving birth when these muscles have been stretched.

Your PF is a hammock of muscles, ligaments and sheet-like tissues that run from your pubic bone to the base of your spine. It supports your bladder, uterus and bowel. If you've ever had a little wee when skipping, coughing or sneezing, then you need to work on your PF. An additional bonus to having a strong PF is that it can increase sensitivity and make sex more satisfying.

Your TVA, the deepest of your core muscles, functions like a corset around your waist. Having a strong TVA is important as it protects the spine by distributing the stresses of bearing weight, thereby preventing injury and reducing the risk of lower back pain.

We're all super busy doing everyday stuff whilst we're sitting down, such as emailing, reading, driving, eating or watching TV. This might lead you to develop slouched shoulders, a hunched back or a generally bad posture. Rather than simply accepting this as a consequence of modern-day life, see it as an opportunity to develop your core as the foundation for strength. Your core is essential for balance and coordination. Core strength also helps you stay mentally strong. And when you are feeling strong and capable, life's obstacles seem a lot easier to tackle.

Sitting up straight is one of the simplest but most effective ways to improve your core strength. The act of sitting up straight immediately engages your core muscles. You grow taller, your stomach is drawn in and instantly flattens, your shoulders are gently pulled back and down. To maintain good posture you need a balance of strength and an awareness of your body – something you may have to constantly remind yourself of until it becomes second nature. It may feel awkward, even a little uncomfortable, at first. But stick with it, your body and muscles are now engaged and working.

*Here are some tips to help you find and
practise good posture:*

Sitting

Keep your legs uncrossed and your feet flat on the
floor. Your weight should be distributed evenly
between your feet, thighs, hips and lower back.

If you can, adjust your chair so your hips are slightly
higher than your knees.

Draw in your navel towards your spine; your abs
should be firm but not too tight.

Keep your shoulders open, relaxed and drawing down
your spine.

Make sure your ears are over your shoulders and don't
allow your chin to push forward.

Never sit for too long. Always take a break and walk
around, which helps to prevent your hamstrings and
lower back from tightening up, which can pull your
spine out of alignment.

Try sitting on a Swiss ball rather than a chair while
working.

Standing

Stand with your feet slightly apart and gently rock
back and forth so you feel the weight of your body
moving from your heels to your toes. Stop when you
feel the weight is evenly distributed over both feet.

Soften your knees and gently draw in your navel
towards your spine, keeping it firm but not too tight.

Keep your shoulders open, relaxed and drawing down
your spine.

Make sure your ears are over your shoulders.

Imagine a line running from your earlobe through
your shoulder, hip, knee and ankle.

In a nutshell

Back straight, shoulders squared, chin level, chest out,
stomach in! Try making these small simple corrections
to the way you sit and stand and see how your body
changes. You are taller, your stomach is flatter, and your
boobs seem bigger. OK, so that's on the vanity side, but
there are other reasons for developing good posture:

To help an aching back, neck, hips or knees.

To prevent injury when exercising.

To slow down or prevent the development of arthritis
and osteoporosis.

To boost confidence, self-esteem, and provide a sense of
empowerment.

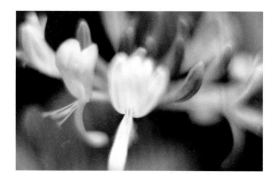

TO MAINTAIN GOOD POSTURE
YOU NEED A BALANCE OF
STRENGTH AND AN AWARENESS
OF YOUR BODY.

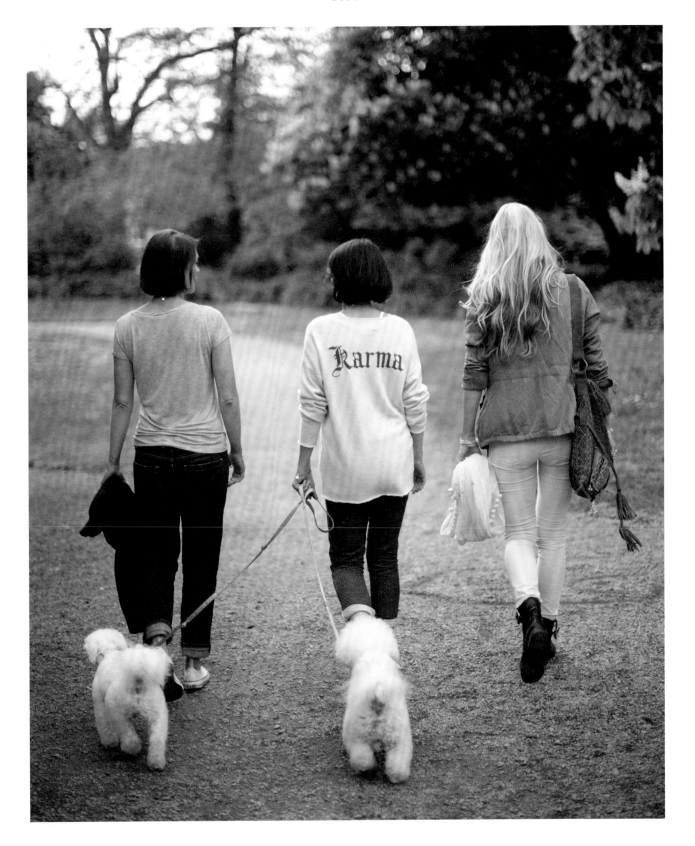

MEASURE ME UP, BABY

It's a great idea to have weekly challenges to push you out of your comfort zone. Do something you haven't done before: run further, skip longer, lift heavier weights, hold the plank position for your longest time yet, and when you feel you've reached your limits, go that little bit further.

Set yourself goals. You need to have a clear idea of what you want to achieve from your exercise routine, and map it out. Think about what you would like to achieve in a year's time and then break this down into smaller targets to reach over the coming months. Writing down your plan shows commitment and it helps to make your goals real.

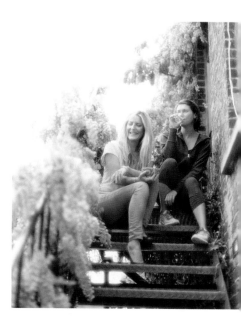

Not all of your goals have to be exercise-related. Having daily targets is a great start and really works for me and for my clients. Pick five things you would like to improve or change for the next week and write them on the action plan. Give yourself a realistic target for how many times that week you are going to achieve your chosen goal. Each day give yourself a tick when you've done it. Likely examples to try for one week might be:

GOAL	TARGET
Drink more water	1.5 litres every day
Exercise regularly	3 times a week for 45 minutes each
Avoid alcohol	5 days this week
Get more sleep	Sleep for at least 7 hours every night
Vary my cooking	Try three new healthy recipes

Fuel your body

It is best to eat within an hour of exercising. Your metabolism is fired up and your body wants some protein and nutritious food to feed your hungry muscles and speed recovery. The hour after exercise is going to be the most beneficial. If you know it's going to be hard to prepare something in that time, then make sure you have a healthy snack to hand. Eat something high in protein to aid in muscle repair: eggs, fish, seeds and nuts are all great sources.

Your body is a furnace

When you exercise for short bursts at a higher intensity you create the after-burn effect which causes your body to burn more calories long after you have stopped exercising. Don't make your workout a punishment for eating badly. Eating a packet of biscuits because you are going to the gym later to 'burn it off' isn't a healthy way to think. Being active and moving your body is an amazing gift of health you give to yourself, exercise is the reward.

Motivate yourself

Too often we get stuck on losing weight, but jumping on the scales every day to see whether the numbers are changing can be a massively disheartening experience, especially if you don't see those numbers going down. It's also pretty stressful and stress equals more cortisol (the stress hormone), which actually holds onto body fat. Think about fat loss, not weight loss. Focus on changing your body shape and don't get obsessed about your weight. Remember that muscle weighs the same as fat. A pound is a pound, right? But a pound of muscle is far more compact – nearly 3 times smaller than fat – so takes up much less space. So if you are 10 stone of lean muscle you are going to look a lot better than if you are 10 stone of fat. It's not about numbers on the scales.

Another myth is that fat turns into muscle. Fat cells can't change into muscle cells. But what you can do is burn fat and build muscle. Body fat is a storage place for extra energy when we consume more calories than we burn. Continue to do this and your fat cells increase in size. When we 'burn fat' what we are doing is shrinking our fat cells. What's good to remember is that the body burns more calories maintaining muscles than it does maintaining fat. So it's time to get strong.

The jeans test

So ditch the scales and grab two pairs of jeans or two of your favourite dresses. The first pair should be a bit snug, the ones you will only pull out when you are feeling super body confident. These will be your go-to test jeans over the first few weeks of your lifestyle change. Each week, slip them on and see how they feel. Remember things don't happen overnight. The second pair of jeans (or dress number two) should be super tight. You know these jeans, we all have them. It's the pair you've kept for years at the back of your wardrobe, hoping one day to hop back into them. These are your 3-month target jeans. It's good to set yourself longer targets to track against your weekly goals so you can see and appreciate the results.

Measure me up, baby

Taking measurements of your body is also a good idea to really 'measure' results. Make a note of them and hide them away. Come back to them every four weeks and record your new measurements. To keep the measurements accurate, take them on exactly the same body part each time and in the same conditions. You might find it easier to get someone to help you. Wear fitted clothes or nothing at all and use a cloth measuring tape.

Arms: Measure the thickest part of your arm (usually around the bicep).

Bust: Place the measuring tape across your nipples and take the largest measurement around your chest keeping the tape parallel to the floor.

Hips: Place the measuring tape around the widest part of your hips/butt, which is usually just above your crotch.

Waist: Place the measuring tape an inch above your belly button (the narrowest part of your waist). Take the measurement after an exhale of breath. Don't suck in your tummy.

Upper thigh: Measure around the widest part of the thigh – usually about three-quarters the way up from your knee.

CARDIO & WEIGHTS

When you exercise for short bursts at a higher intensity you create the afterburn effect, also known as EPOC (excess post-exercise oxygen consumption). This causes your body to continue to burn a higher number of calories long after you have stopped exercising. Sounds great!! Really? Yes! So by working harder for shorter bursts of time, overall you burn more calories.

If you are training for a distance run, then obviously running for a long period of time is going to benefit your training and help you reach your goal. But if you are trying to lose weight, don't spend hours on the treadmill or cross trainer; stop watching the numbers to see how many calories you have burned. You need to mix it up and HIIT (high intensity interval training – see page 242) it! Using the HIIT method shocks your body and ramps up your metabolism for fat loss. Push yourself out of your usual comfort zone for as little as only 3 minutes. Go faster for short bursts. For example, ride the stationary bike for 3 minutes, going as fast as you can for 30 seconds, then slowing down to catch your breath for 30 seconds, repeat until you've done the fast and slower cycles each 3 times. You will get fitter and see great results while taking only a quarter of the time.

Doing the same cardio routine can get boring so keep it varied and find something you enjoy – cycling, swimming or hiking perhaps. It doesn't have to mean slogging away on a treadmill. There are so many body weight exercises that really get your heart rate up, such as skipping, squat thrusts, mountain climbers and burpees.

BECOME MORE CONFIDENT. WHEN YOUR BODY IS STRONG IT POSITIVELY AFFECTS OTHER AREAS IN YOUR LIFE.

You won't get bulky

There is fear in a lot of women that if you use heavy weights you will create a big and bulky unfeminine body. I can tell you right now this is NOT true. What is bulky is fat! Lifting weights will create a leaner, more athletic, elegant-looking body.

There is one simple reason why women can't acquire muscle mass to the same degree as men and it's down to the hormone testosterone. Women only produce a tiny amount of this hormone; men will produce roughly 20 times more. Even taking that into account, creating muscle in men still isn't easy and takes a huge amount of hard work and dedication. So don't be scared of lifting heavy weights – this is the key to making real changes to your body shape.

Top reasons why women should lift weights

Increases your metabolism and basal metabolic rate (BMR) so your body burns more calories each day

Reduces the chance of osteoporosis by increasing bone density

Tones and sculpts your body and gives it definition by increasing muscle tissue

Releases the happy hormone so your mood and energy levels increase, which in turn reduces anxiety and depression

Keeps you young – it's the most effective anti-ageing activity

Reduces many lifestyle-related diseases and chronic illnesses

Increases quality of life and well-being overall

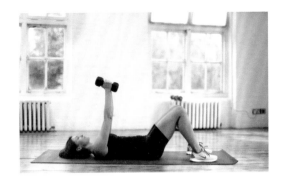

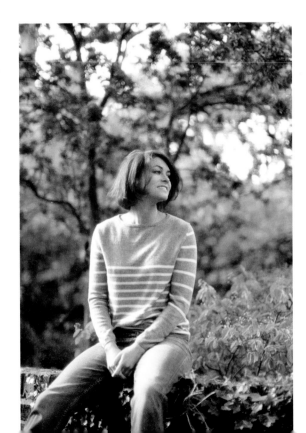

EXERCISE
THROUGH *the* YEARS

20s

Your body is pretty strong in your 20s and can take the abuse of excessive parties, binge drinking and bad eating habits. But that doesn't mean we can't still give our bodies some TLC. Your 20s is the decade in which to build your base fitness and create habits for a lifetime. Think of your body as a bank of goodness: start paying in early and your body will repay you in later years.

30s

Mix up your training. If you stuck to one sport in your early years, now is a good time to cross-train by adding something new. Staying with one thing over a long period also causes postural imbalances whereas working a variety of muscles will help prevent injury. You might find it harder to shift those unwanted pounds in your 30s, as with each decade our metabolic base rate drops by 1–2 per cent. If you have exercised regularly and kept a healthy lifestyle you won't see that big a difference in your body shape. Remember your body bank and keep paying those installments.

40s

Preserve your strength and fight belly fat. Now is the time to increase your weight lifting. In your 40s, your body begins to lose muscle mass. By lifting weights you will preserve your lean muscle mass, which will keep your metabolic rate high so you continue to burn optimum calories. Gravity, hormones and your slowing metabolism are a triple hit in this decade and you may find it harder to see results. But by keeping your exercise routine consistent with cardio and resistance training, you will keep your muscle mass.

50s

Your heart and core are key in this decade. Aches and pains are likely to crop up in your 50s, but don't be put off. Adapt your exercise to work with your body not against it – there is always something you can do. Pilates and yoga are great ways to strengthen your core and keep your posture from slouching. And good posture is not only vital for your health, it helps you look young. Keep your heart strong by doing at least 30 minutes of moderate exercise 4–5 times a week.

60s

This decade is about prevention. Keeping your exercise up now is super important. You should be lifting weights two or three times a week. A simple weight training resistance programme protects you from the slippery slope of frailty and helps prevent falls. Any break or fracture will take much longer to heal so your balance is a good thing to focus on. As your joints and ligaments start to become stiffer, add more stretches. If you haven't tried yoga, it can be a lovely gentle way to keep your body mobile and flexible.

70s

Young at heart and still raring to go, walking isn't the only exercise you can do in your 70s. Keep it varied and work on balance, flexibility and strength. And continue to do the things you enjoy.

80s, 90s, 100s

There is never a cut-off point, keep active forever. Whatever your age, it's not too late to start exercising. Take it slowly and never work through pain.

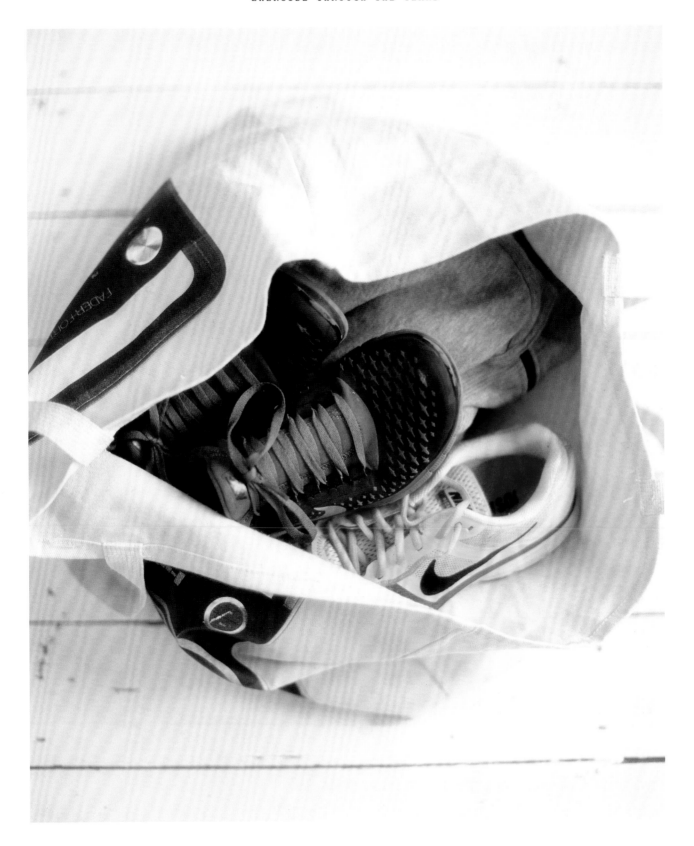

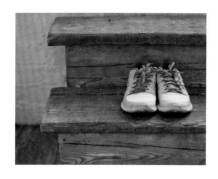

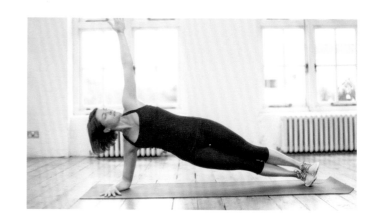

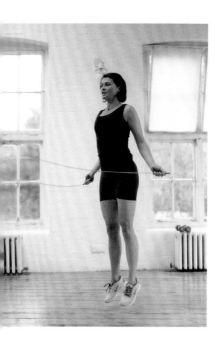

your

FOUR WEEK EXERCISE

programme

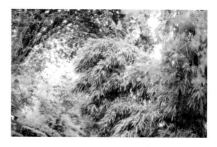

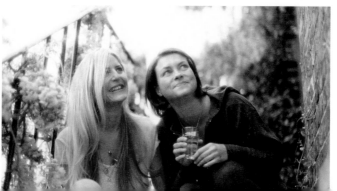

The programmes I have created use functional exercises that imitate your daily activities. The aim is to make you stronger so your life gets easier and you can go about your daily tasks without risking injury. When you are not exercising, your daily routine still requires you to move – balancing, twisting, bending, pulling, pushing are all part of everyday life, whether it's lifting your children, carrying heavy shopping, or pushing the vacuum cleaner. I am not in favour of using gym machines because they make your body perform an exercise that restricts it to a certain movement, and that isn't how your body naturally moves. Learning how to do functional exercise correctly will lead to better joint mobility and general stability (a client once told me how happy she was that after exercising and learning to control her body she could now stand on the tube without having to hold on for dear life because her balance was so improved).

Variation is key to my clients' success and that's what I have developed here: full body workouts that progress as the weeks pass but are never repeated. Your body and mind are always kept guessing and being challenged in different ways. There is nothing worse than doing the same thing week in, week out.

LET'S BEGIN

You will need:
- Gymboss app or timer
- Skipping rope: this is my favourite bit of kit. Cheap, compact and amazing for a cardio blast. Get a plastic or nylon one
- Dumbbells: choose ones that weigh between 3 and 6kg
- Swiss ball: this inflatable ball can double up as a chair and is great for your posture
- A mat or even just a room with a soft carpet.

Foam roller

A bonus piece of kit I love. You can use a foam roller to help warm up your muscles before a workout or to lengthen tight muscles post-workout. By rolling your body over the roller you break down adhesions between the muscle fibres, allowing more blood to pump through your body. Rather like a deep tissue massage, it can be quite painful to begin with. It's great for getting those hard to reach spots like your IT band (the tendon that runs from your hip to the outside of your knee).

Tips when using the roller
- Stay on the soft tissue and don't roll over bone or joints
- Roll over each area at least 10 times
- If you hit a really painful spot it's probably a trigger point. Hold for a few seconds and allow the muscle to release

Warm Up

Any exercise programme must be preceded by a warm up and followed by a stretch (see page 208) to ensure you avoid injury. Warming up gradually increases the circulation of oxygen to your muscles, heart and lungs, making your work out more effective. It is also a good opportunity to visualise your goals and focus on how great you will feel when you achieve them.

Complete the following movements one after the other for 20 seconds each. You're aiming to raise your heart rate as you warm up, so by the end you should feel slightly out of breath with your mind and body ready for exercise. The warm up should take 3 minutes.

CREATING YOUR OWN WORKOUT SPACE IS A GREAT IDEA. THAT WAY, IF YOU DON'T HAVE ACCESS TO A GYM OR ARE SHORT OF TIME YOU ARE ALWAYS PREPARED FOR A HOME WORKOUT SESSION.

09

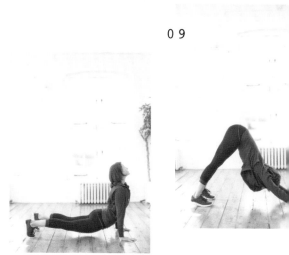

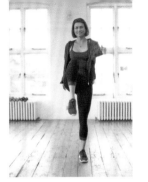
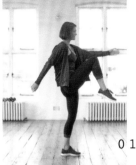

01

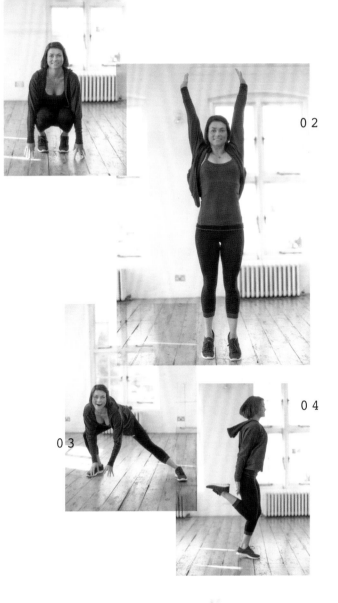

02

04

03

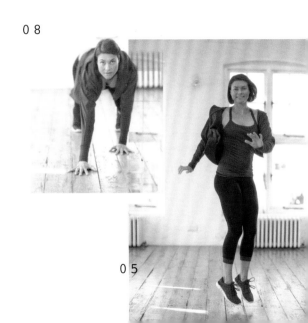

08

05

01 March
Bring your knees to your chest in a marching action.

02 Down and up
Crouch down and touch the floor, heels raised, then stand up onto your tiptoes and reach for the ceiling.

03 Lunge with side step
Start in a standing position and bend into a side lunge, step back to standing and then repeat on the other side.

04 Butt kicks
Hopping from one leg to the other, bring your heel up to your butt.

05 Jumping twist
Jump whilst rotating your upper and lower body in different directions.

06 Shoulder windmills
With straight arms, rotate them both backwards in big circles; repeat in a forwards rotation.

07 Fast jog and punch
Jogging on the spot doing a fast forward punching action.

08 Caterpillar
From a standing position, place both hands on the floor and walk them forward to a plank, walk them back and return to a standing position.

09 Downward and upward facing dog
Move in a flowing motion from one position to the next.

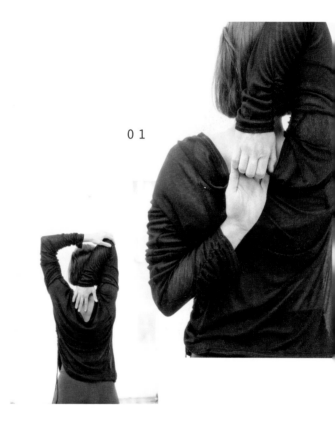

01

Stretch

Just as you need to warm up at the start of each
workout, you should also stretch at the end. Taking
the time to stretch is one of the most important parts
of a workout. It provides the opportunity to relax the
mind as well as the body. Picturing the muscle you are
stretching and breathing 'into that area' will help to
relax and relieve it further.

Stretching also helps to lengthen and open your body,
releasing any tension in the muscles after exercise.

**Hold each stretch for 20 seconds, just at the point
where it begins to feel uncomfortable. Use your
breathing to relax into the stretch, inhaling and
exhaling deeply. This series of stretches should take
4–5 minutes.**

01 **Triceps stretch** – straighten one arm up towards the
ceiling, then bend it at the elbow taking your hand down
the centre of your spine. With the other hand, gently
pull the elbow behind your head. To increase the stretch
interlace your fingers. Repeat on the other side.

02 **Chest and shoulder opener** – interlace your hands
behind your back. Lift your straight arms away from your
back. If you can, squeeze the palms of your hands together.

03 **Cat and Cow** – to stretch and open your spine. Start
on all fours and slowly move from photo 03a to 03b; move
fluidly for 20 seconds.

04 **Downward facing dog** – a wonderful full body stretch,
especially good for your hamstrings. Press your heels
towards the floor and then alternate heel press.

05 **Pigeon pose** – start on all fours, bring your right knee
to your right wrist, straighten your back leg and lower

yourself down so your right ankle is below your left hip. To
increase the stretch lower your head to the floor. Repeat on
the other side.

06 **Seated spinal twist** – sit on the floor with your knees
bent, slide your right foot under your left leg, placing your
right foot by your left hip. Step your left foot over the right
leg and place it by your right knee. Twist towards your bent
knee. Repeat on the other side.

07 **Hip flexor stretch** – with your left knee pressing
slightly into the floor, tuck your tailbone under and gently
push your hip forward. Be careful not to sink down too
deeply. To increase the stretch raise your left arm and bend
gently to the right. Repeat on the other side.

08 **Quad stretch** – from your hip flexor stretch position,
reach back and pick up your back ankle, bring your foot
towards your butt. Repeat on the other side.

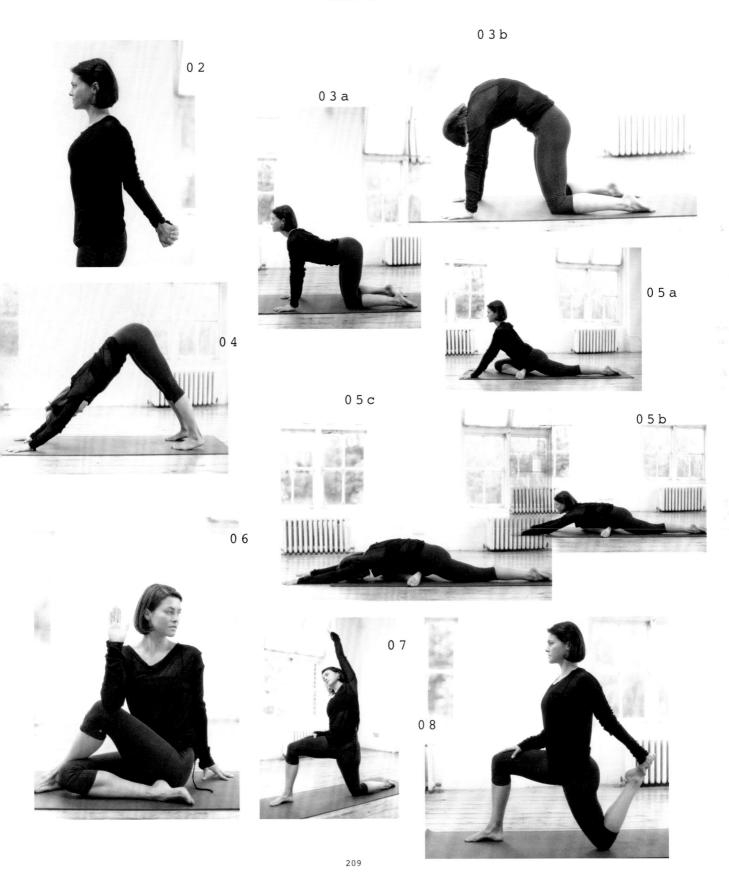

0 2

0 3 b

0 3 a

0 4

0 5 a

0 5 c

0 5 b

0 6

0 7

0 8

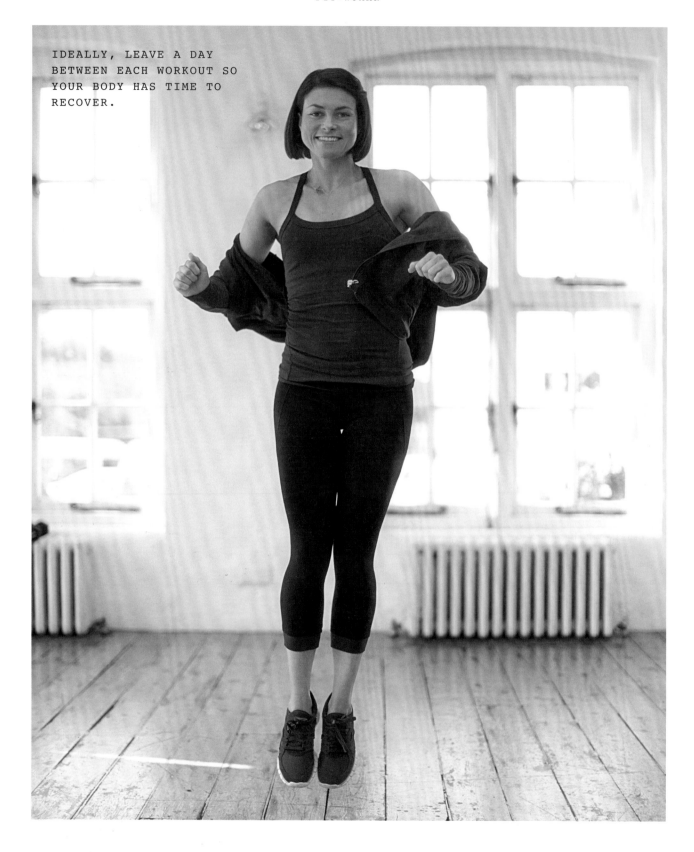

IDEALLY, LEAVE A DAY
BETWEEN EACH WORKOUT SO
YOUR BODY HAS TIME TO
RECOVER.

WEEK ONE

get moving

Timing
30 seconds on each exercise
15 seconds between exercises
Repeat circuit 3 times
90 seconds rest between each circuit

Tips for the week ahead

Workout 1

Make sure you get ready for the week, plan your workouts now and know which days you're training. Have a plan B in place just in case.

Get a good sports bra. Protect your boobs, ladies. Seriously, bouncing up and down can be not only painful but also it can stretch the tissue around your bust. Chest exercises will give you a boob lift, so don't undo all that good work.

Skipping – don't put too much pressure on yourself to get it right the first time. Just give it a go and see what happens! If it's driving you crazy and you can't get it then drop the rope and continue to skip with an imaginary rope.

Cardio is any form of exercise that increases your heart rate.

If you're finding things tough don't worry, we all had to start somewhere and it gets easier, I promise you! Complete the workout at your own pace, congratulate yourself for however much you achieve today.

Workout 2

Squats are one of the best all-round exercises targeting the biggest muscles – your butt and thighs – plus they activate your core and pretty much every other muscle in your lower body. Serious fat burn. Learn to love your squats.

Feeling a bit achy today? That's normal – it just means that you worked hard. Drink plenty of water and follow the stretches at the end of each workout. It's a great time to have a magnesium bath – this essential mineral will go straight to help your aching muscles recover quickly. I love the magnesium bath soak from betteryou.uk.com.

Healthy snacks for the handbag: Amber's Coconut & Apricot Bliss Balls (page 91), almonds, oatcakes, apples. Don't eat them all at once, though!

Today's motto: I don't FIND the time to exercise, I MAKE the time to exercise – try saying it out loud.

Workout 3

Brace your core and engage your stomach muscles. Imagine you are about to be punched in the stomach (not a very nice thought but it works!). Be sure to keep them tight throughout the whole exercise – and remember to breathe!

Remember this is a lifestyle change, so start replacing bad habits with good ones.

Mini challenge – did you know that lean muscle is 80 per cent water? If you become dehydrated your muscles won't contract properly. Give yourself the H_2O challenge today and drink at least 1 litre of water. Try adding cucumber or lemon for that extra freshness.

How do I zip up my pelvic floor? Imagine your pelvic floor is the slider of a zip, being zipped up as you lift your butt. Squeeze from the back (inside your butt) to your navel. Using visualisations like this can really help.

Week One

WORKOUT 1

3–5 minute warm up

01 **Alternating lunge**
Thighs, butt, core
- Stand with your feet hip width apart, hands on hips.
- Take a big step forward bending both knees; your front knee should not extend beyond your toes.
- As your back knee almost touches the floor push back to the start and alternate legs.
- Engage your core to keep your balance throughout this move.

02 **Dips with bent knees**
Triceps, core, 'bingo wings'
- Come to the edge of a chair, fingers facing forward.
- With your knees bent lower your body, bending your elbows to 90 degrees and push back up.
- Keep your back close to the chair throughout.

03 **Jogging on spot with arms raised**
Cardio, fat burn
- Raise both arms above your head.
- Jog on the spot bringing your knees up as high as you can, lifting your feet off the ground.

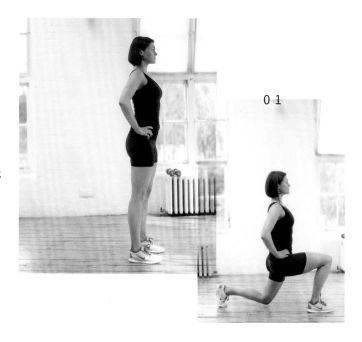

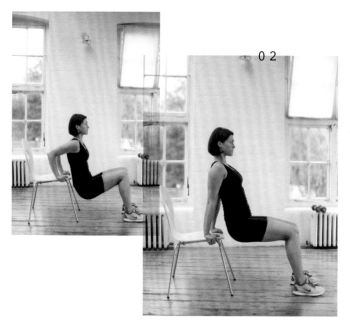

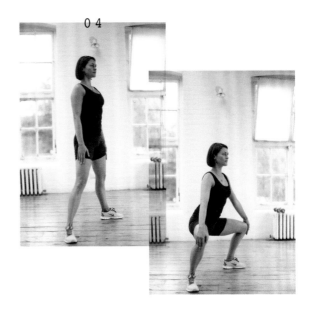

04 **Plié squat**
Inner thigh, butt, core
- Stand with your feet wider than shoulder width apart – toes pointing out (second position for any ballerinas out there).
- With your back straight, lower your body so your knees are in line with your toes.
- Push through your heels back up to starting position.
- Remember to keep your shoulders back, engaging your core, abs, and pelvic floor.

05 **Kneeling press up**
Chest, shoulders, triceps, core
- Get on all fours.
- Walk your hands forward one hand space.
- Shift your weight forward so your shoulders are over your hands.
- Bend your arms with your elbows pointing backwards and lower your body.
- As your chest almost touches the floor, push up back to the starting position.
- Keep your head in line with your body throughout.

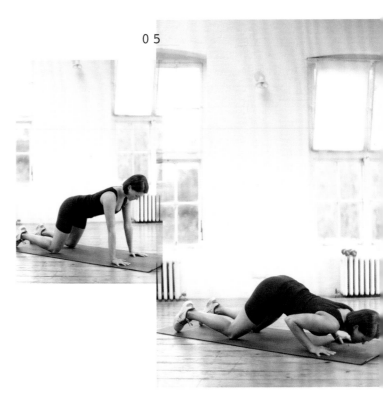

06 **Skipping**
Cardio, fat burn
- Hold the skipping rope handles at hip level with the rope on the floor behind you.
- Flick your wrists and swing the rope over your head.
- Just before it hits the floor jump, keeping both feet together.

To finish
4 minute stretch

Week One

WORKOUT 2

3–5 minute warm up

01 Side lunge

Inner thigh, outer thigh, butt, core

- Stand tall with your back nice and straight.
- Take a big step to one side.
- Bend your landing leg to 90 degrees.
- Push your hips back, keeping your bent knee over your ankle.
- With a big push, come back up to standing and repeat on the other side.

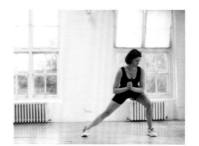
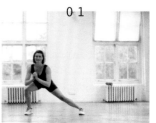

02 Arm curl to shoulder press

Biceps, shoulders, core

- Stand with your feet hip width apart and with a slight soft bend in the knees.
- Hold the weights at your sides and engage your core.
- With your palms facing upwards, curl the weights up to your shoulders.
- Open your arms out so your palms now face forward.
- Press the weights from your shoulders to above your head.
- Slowly reverse the move back through the curl.

03 Squats

Thighs, butt, core

- Stand tall with your feet shoulder width apart. You can place an exercise ball behind you if you wish (as shown).
- Hold your arms straight out in front of you at shoulder height.
- Keep your back straight and bend your knees until your butt just touches the ball.
- Push your hips back and keep your weight over your heels.
- Stand back up and repeat.

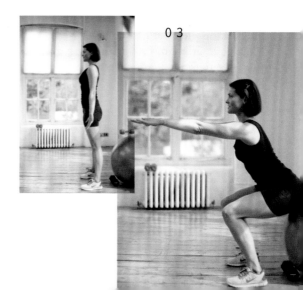

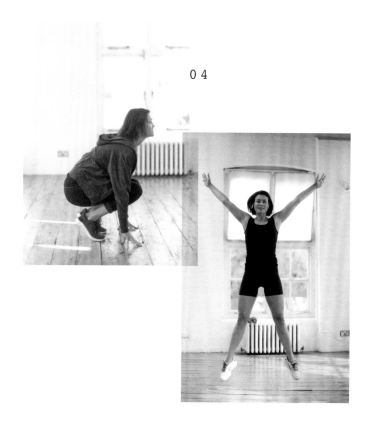

04 **Jumping Jacks**
Cardio, fat burn
- Start with your feet together, crouch down and bend at the knees so your fingers can touch the floor.
- Jump up and spread out your arms and legs to form an X shape.
- Jump straight back down into your crouch position and repeat.

05 **Back raise**
Upper back, shoulders
- Lie down on your front.
- Spread out your arms so you are making a T shape, palms facing down.
- With your thumbs up, raise your arms and upper body off the floor; arching your upper back slightly.
- Pause and slowly lower yourself back down to the starting position.
- Don't press your stomach into the ground; use your back muscles to raise up.

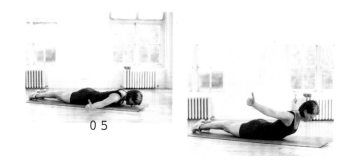

06 **Egg roll**
Abs, core, balance
- Sit upright on the floor.
- Bring your knees towards your body, keeping your feet together and flat on the floor.
- Keeping your hands on your shins, round your back and tuck your tail bone under.
- Roll back onto your shoulders in a nice smooth action, ensuring that you do NOT roll back onto your neck, then roll back to the starting position.

To finish
4 minute stretch

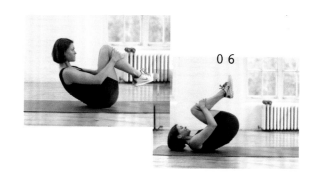

Week One

WORKOUT 3

3–5 minute warm up

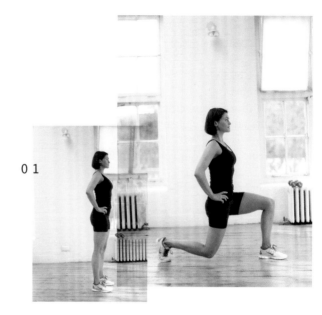

01 **Backward lunge**
Thighs, butt, calves, core
- Stand with your feet hip width apart, with your hands on your hips.
- Take a big step backwards, bending both knees to 90 degrees with the back knee almost touching the floor. Remember to engage your core.
- Push back to the start and repeat, alternating your legs.

02 **Plank with pelvic floor squeeze**
Core, arms
- Get on all fours with your hands under your shoulders.
- Straighten your legs, pushing your heels back.
- You should now be in a nice straight line from head to ankles.
- Brace your core, keeping your body firm, and squeeze your pelvic floor (see tip on page 211).

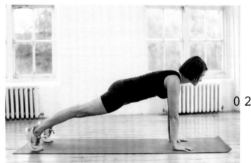

03 **Flies on the floor**
Chest, core
- Lie on your back with your knees bent and your feet hip width apart.
- Grab a weight in each hand and hold them above you in line with your shoulders, palms facing each other.
- Engage your core and slightly bend your arms.
- Lower your arms to an inch away from touching the floor. Pause and return to the start position.

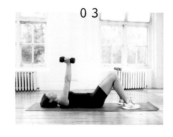
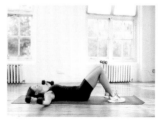

04 **Hips raised bridge with pelvic floor squeezes**
Back, butt, thighs, core
- Lie on your back with your knees bent and your feet hip width apart.
- Engage your stomach muscles and 'zip up' your pelvic floor.
- Push your heels into the floor to raise your hips.
- Your body should be in a straight line from your shoulders to your knees.
- Hold this position and squeeze and release your pelvic floor.

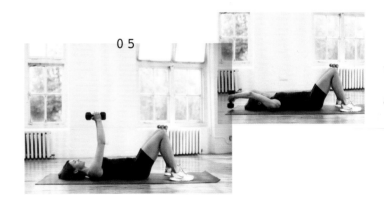

05 **Single dumb-bell pullover**
Back, arms, core
- Lie on your back with your knees bent and your feet hip width apart.
- Hold one weight straight above you with both hands and engage your stomach muscles.
- With a slight bend in your elbows, lower the weight back over your head towards the floor.
- When the weight is an inch or so from the floor, pause and lift back to the start position.

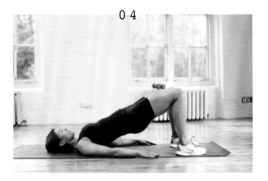

06 **Skipping**
Cardio, fat burn
- Hold the skipping rope handles at hip level with the rope on the floor behind you.
- Flick your wrists and swing the rope over your head.
- Just before it hits the floor jump, keeping both feet together.

To finish
4 minute stretch

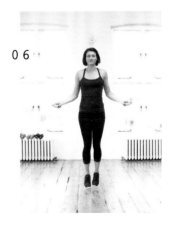

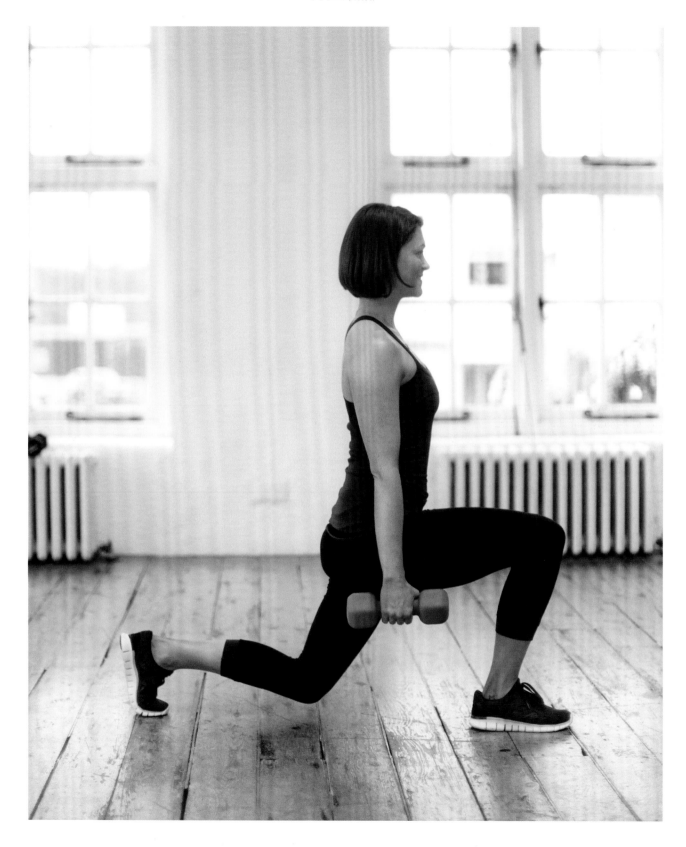

WEEK TWO

get strong

Timing

40 seconds on each exercise
15 seconds between exercises
Repeat circuit 3 times
90 seconds rest between each circuit

Tips for the week ahead

Workout 1

Be proud of the changes you are making, no matter how small, and don't forget the value of a workout. It's about how it makes you feel, not just how many calories you burn.

Cardio HIT! Smash it girls and give it everything! Getting your heart rate up for short bursts maximises your fat-burn and is great for fitness.

Let's go nuts. Walnuts contain more antioxidants, folic acid and vitamin E than any other nut, plus you get your essential omega 3 fats. Tasty too!

Workout 2

The SOS wave (page 222) is for balance. It's a body and mind exercise to focus on your core, coordination and concentration. When these three are top of their game, your workouts will be accelerated.

Think of getting enough sleep as being just as important as eating a healthy diet and getting regular exercise. Getting 7 hours of sleep after a day of healthy eating and moderate exercise can lower the risk of heart disease by up to 65 per cent.

Mini challenger: try getting 7 hours sleep tonight.

Workout 3

Have you got that Friday feeling? Remember, everything in moderation, don't wake up with a hangover tomorrow, you know you'll regret it.

Don't make excuses for why you can't get your exercise done. Focus on all the reasons why you must make it happen.

Halfway there, well done! Set your goals and targets for next week. Write them down, tell someone about them. Make them real and make them happen.

Week Two

WORKOUT 1

3–5 minute warm up

01 **Backward lunge with knee raise
(20 seconds each side)**
Thighs, calves, core, butt, balance
• Stand tall with your feet hip width apart.
• Take a big step backward, bending both knees to
90 degrees with the back knee almost touching the
floor. Remember to engage your core.
• With a big push off the back foot, drive your back
knee up towards your chest.
• Take the lifted leg straight back into the backward
lunge position and repeat.

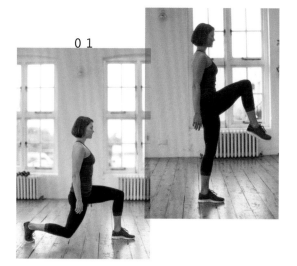

02 **Mountain climbers**
Cardio, fat burn, core, legs, shoulders
• Get into a high plank position with your shoulders
above your hands and your heels pushing back.
• Keep your body in a straight line from your head to
your heels – no high butts please.
• Bring one knee towards your chest and tap your toe
to the floor.
• Moving quickly, repeat with the other leg and
continue alternating.
• Keep your stomach muscles engaged throughout to
feel the burn.

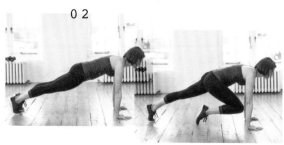

03 **Triceps kick back**
Triceps, core
• Grab your weights and stand with your feet hip
width apart, knees slightly bent.
• Engage your core and lean forward from the hips so
your butt sticks out, with your arms by your sides
and elbows bent.
• Keeping your elbows close to your body, straighten
your arms back behind you.
• Pause and squeeze your triceps (the muscle on the
back of your arm).
• Bring your arms back to the start and repeat.

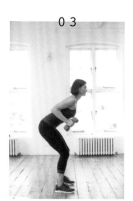
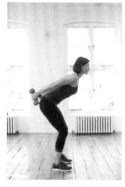

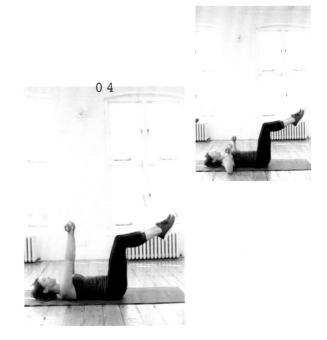

04 **Chest press with table top legs**
Chest, triceps, core
- Grab your weights in each hand and lie on your back, feet off the ground and knees in line with your hips.
- Gently press your back into the floor and engage your stomach muscles.
- Hold the weights straight above you in line with your shoulders and palms away.
- Bend your elbows and lower the weights until your arms touch the floor (elbows at 90 degrees).
- Push back up into the start position and repeat.

05 **Superman with pelvic floor squeeze (20 seconds per leg and arm)**
Butt, back, core, pelvic floor
- Get on all fours, hands under your shoulders and knees under your hips.
- Keep your back flat and your stomach muscles engaged.
- Straighten your left leg back behind you and raise it so your ankle is in line with your hip, so you have a straight line from your head to your ankle.
- Squeeze your butt as you lift your leg.
- At the same time raise your right arm straight out in front of you.
- Return back to all fours, and repeat.

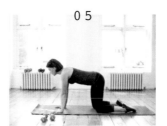
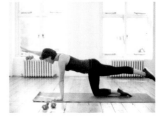

06 **Modified squat thrust on Swiss ball against a wall**
Cardio, fat burn, core, leg, shoulders
- Place a Swiss ball against a wall and get into the plank position with your hands on the Swiss ball.
- Engage your stomach muscles, creating a strong core.
- Jump your feet in towards your chest and straight back out to the starting position and repeat.
- Keep your core engaged and your butt down throughout.

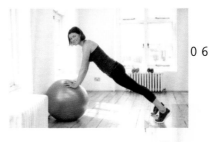
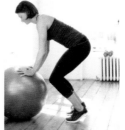

To finish
4 minute stretch

Week Two

WORKOUT 2

3–5 minute warm up

01 Walking lunge with weights
Thighs, butt, core
- Stand with your feet hip width apart, holding your weights by your sides.
- Take a big step forward and bend both knees; your front knee shouldn't extend beyond your toe.
- As your back knee almost touches the floor, push off your back foot and take a big step forward, bending both knees.
- Keep your core engaged to help with balance and use the length of your room to walk your lunges forward.

02 Skipping
Cardio, fat burn
- Just as we did in Week One (see page 217).
- If you feel ready, try to pick up the speed.
- Move onto a single jump.

03 Single leg balance with SOS wave (20 seconds per leg)
Core, balance, upper back, shoulders
- Stand tall with your feet hip width apart with your arms by your sides, palms facing forward.
- Find a spot at eye level to focus on.
- Engage your core and shift your weight onto your left leg.
- Bend your right leg and raise your knee to your chest as high as you can.
- Keeping good balance, slowly lift your arms away from your sides and above your head, squeezing your shoulder blades. Repeat, alternating legs.

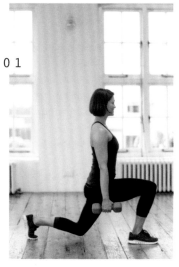

01

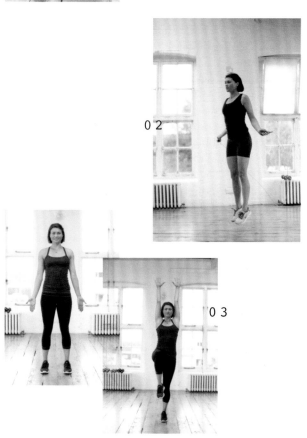

02

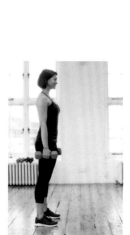

03

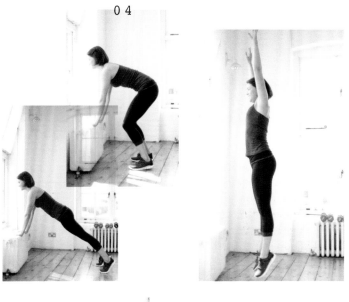

04 **Modified burpee (squat thrust with jump)**
Cardio, fat burn, core, legs
• Start with your hands on a chair or a step (the higher you are, the easier you are making it) and keep your legs straight back behind you.
• Engage your core and keep your abs tight throughout.
• You should be in a straight line from head to ankles as in a high plank.
• Don't let your hips drop down.
• Jump both feet towards your chest and take the weight in your legs.
• From here jump straight up reaching your arms in the air.
• Once landed return back to start position and repeat.

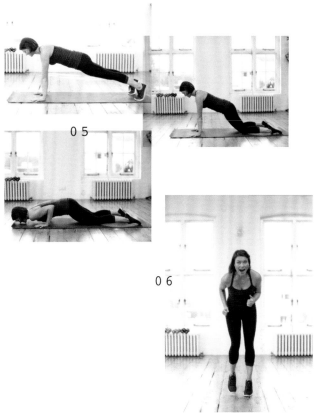

05 **Kneeling press ups**
(as in Week One, Workout 1, but more challenging)
Chest, triceps, core
• Start in a high plank position with your hands under your shoulders.
• Bend your knees and lower to the floor.
• With your elbows facing backwards, lower your body until your chest almost touches the floor.
• Pause at the bottom and push back to the start position.

06 **Fast feet with sprinter's arms**
Cardio, fat burn
• Stand up on the balls of your feet with your knees slightly bent and leaning slightly forward.
• Break into a fast run on the spot.
• Move your arms and feet as fast as you can.
• Imagine a 100m sprint and you are going to win it!

To finish
4 minute stretch

Week two

WORKOUT 3

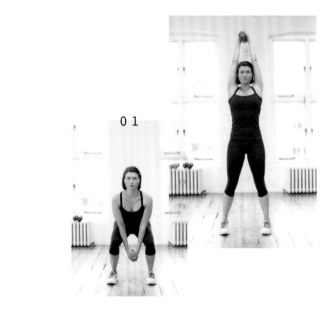

3–5 minute warm up

01 **Dumbbell swing**
Butt, abs, core
- Stand tall with your feet shoulder width apart, holding one weight in front of you with both hands.
- Keeping your back straight, lower into a squat, keeping your body weight in your heels and swinging your weight in front of you.
- Push into your heels and thrust your hips forward as you stand up tall.
- With straight arms swing your weight above your head.
- Make sure your abs are tight and your core is engaged throughout.
- Swing the weight to the start position and repeat, keeping a fluid motion throughout.

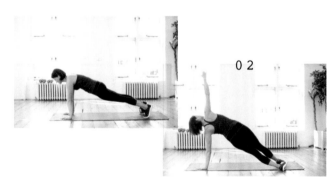

02 **Plank into side arm balance**
Core, waist, shoulders
- Get into a high plank position with your feet hip width apart.
- Keep a straight line from your head to your ankles and your hands beneath your shoulders.
- Reach up to the sky with one hand, turning your body as you do, so that you are balancing in a T shape.
- Bring your arm back to the start position on the floor and repeat on the other side.
- Keep your body straight and your core engaged throughout.

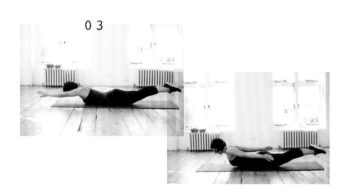

03 **Dry swimming**
Back
- Lie on your front, arms out straight ahead.
- Keeping your legs together, raise them off the floor and hold.
- Raise your chest and arms off the floor and do a breast stroke motion, looking at the floor.
- Don't push your stomach into the floor, make sure your back does the work.

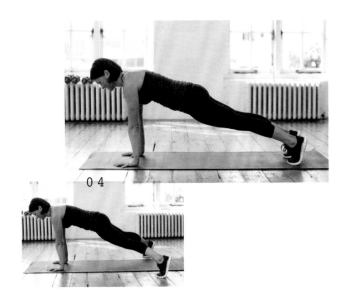

04 **Plank straddle jumps**
Cardio, fat burn, core, abs, shoulders, legs
- Get into a high plank position.
- Keep a straight line from your head to your ankles and your hands beneath your shoulders.
- Keep your core tight and zip up your pelvic floor.
- Jump your legs out wide and then jump them straight back together.
- Don't cheat; keep your butt down throughout.

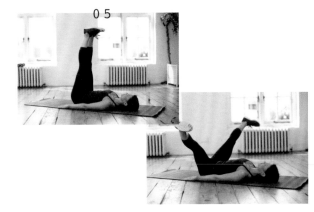

05 **V shaped legs**
Inner thighs, abs, core
- Lie on your back with your feet straight up in the air, feet flexed.
- Slightly press your lower back into the floor and draw your stomach in, engaging your pelvic floor and core.
- Open your legs as wide as you can, pause and slowly bring them back to the start position. Repeat.

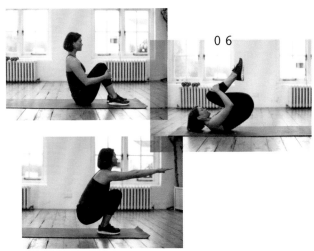

06 **Egg roll**
Core, abs, balance
- Sit upright on the floor.
- Bring your knees towards your body, keeping your feet hip width apart and flat on the floor.
- Keep your hands together on your shins, round your back and tuck your tail bone under.
- Roll back onto your shoulders in a nice smooth action, ensuring you do not roll back onto your neck.
- Roll back to the starting position reaching forward with your arms and trying to raise your butt off the floor. Repeat.

To finish
4 minute stretch

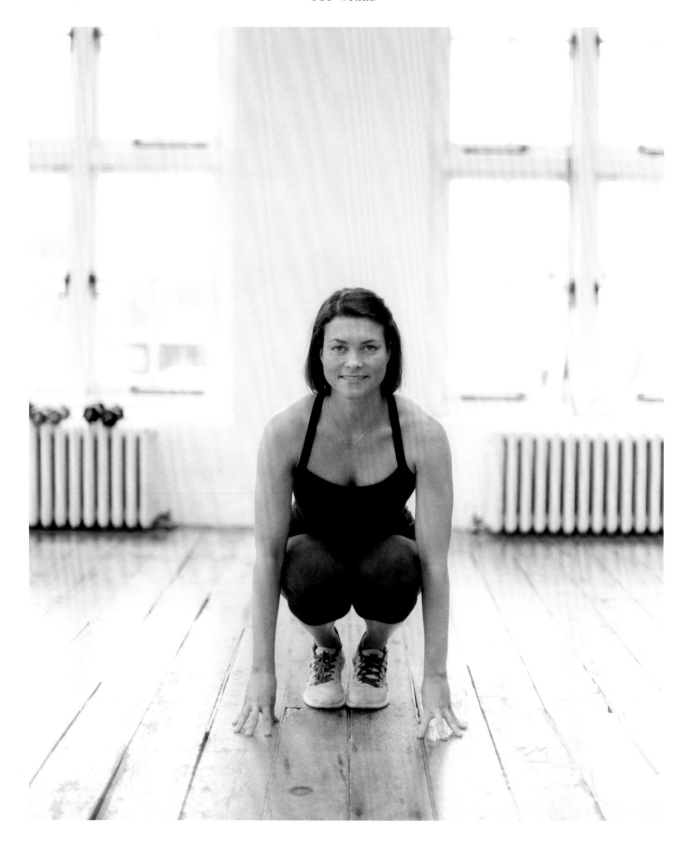

WEEK THREE

get lean

Timing

50 seconds on each exercise
10 seconds between exercises
Repeat circuit 3 times
60 seconds rest between each circuit

Tips for the week ahead

Workout 1

Spending time exercising and strengthening your back is a sure-fire way to have a happy, healthy pain-free back.

Don't ever skip breakfast. It will fire up your metabolism for the day and stop you from grabbing a sugary, fatty snack later on.

Don't think lifting weights is going to bulk you up; think lean and strong. After a workout with weights your metabolism is raised for hours after – meaning you'll still be burning fat while you are sat at your desk!

Workout 2

Make sure you have rest days as these are times for your muscles to repair and heal. Days off are just as important as days on.

High protein meals are what you should have after a workout. Protein goes straight to repair your tissues and is what your body is crying out for. Try Quinoa with a Rainbow of Jewels (page 62) or Baked Pollock (page 76).

When it comes to the Egg roll, don't worry if you spend more time on your butt than on your feet. Keep trying and don't forget to laugh: remember exercise is fun!

Pain in your lower back? Make sure to check your form and focus on engaging you core while you exercise. You should never feel pain in your back or your knees.

Workout 3

A million abdominal crunches won't give you a flat stomach – Russian twists, squats, woodchops, planks and keeping good posture will. And stick to your healthy eating. Bring on that flat stomach!

Bounding, skipping and jumping are all great for increasing bone density.

Week three

WORKOUT 1

3–5 minute warm up

01 Squat thrusts
Cardio, fat burn, core, abs, legs, shoulders
- Assume the high plank position with your arms straight and your shoulders over your hands.
- Engage your stomach muscles creating a nice strong core.
- Jump your feet in towards your chest and straight back out to the starting position and repeat.
- Keep your core engaged throughout and your butt down.

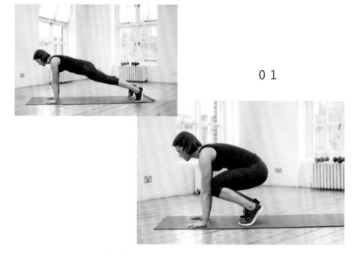

01

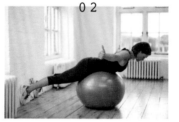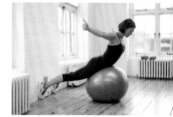

02

02 Thumbs out dorsal raise on Swiss ball
Back, shoulders, balance
- Lie down with your front on a Swiss ball with your toes touching the floor.
- Spread your arms out so you are forming a T shape.
- With your thumbs up, raise your arms and upper body off the Swiss ball, keep your toes on the floor and hips on the ball.
- Pause and slowly lower back to the starting position.

03

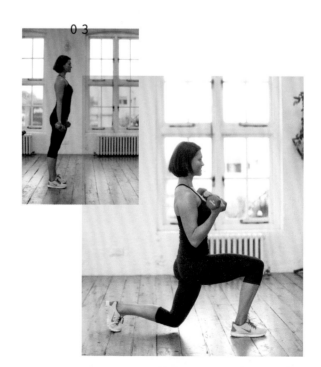

03 Weighted lunge with bicep curl
Thighs, butt, biceps, core
- Grab your weights and stand with your feet hip width apart.
- Hold the weights by your side with your palms facing forward.
- Take a big step forward bending both knees; your front knee should not go beyond your toes.
- As your back knee almost touches the floor, hold the position and curl the weights up towards your shoulders.
- Push back to the start, lowering the weights.
- Repeat, alternating legs.

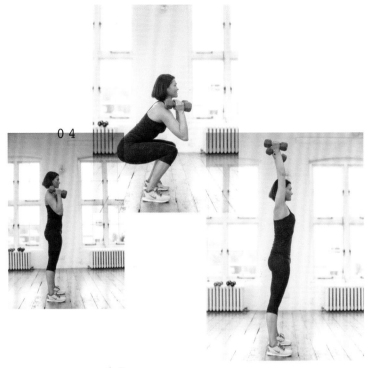

04 **Weighted squat to shoulder press**
Thighs, butt, core, shoulders
- Grab your weights and stand tall, with your feet shoulder width apart.
- Hold your weights at shoulder height with a bent elbow.
- Keep your back straight and bend your knees until your knees are at 90 degrees.
- Push your hips back and keep your weight over your heels.
- Stand back up, lifting the weights above your head as you reach standing position.
- Lower the weights back to shoulder level and repeat.

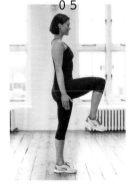
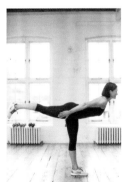

05 **Knee to chest and donkey kick**
(25 seconds each side)
Balance, butt, core
- Stand tall with your feet hip width apart, arms by your side.
- Bring one knee up toward your chest.
- Keeping a straight back, bending from the hip and keeping your arms still, kick your raised leg back behind you, allowing your body to come forward.
- Return to standing position and repeat with the other leg.

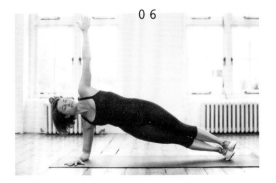

06 **Side plank (25 seconds each side)**
Cardio blast, fat burn, core, leg, shoulders
- Lie on your side.
- Place your elbow directly beneath your shoulder.
- Raise your hips off the ground and reach to the ceiling with your left arm so your body is in a straight line from head to heels.
- After 20 seconds gently lower, turn over and repeat on the other side.

To finish
4 minute stretch

Week three

WORKOUT 2

3–5 minute warm up

01 Elevated back lunge (25 seconds per side)
Thighs, butt, core, balance
• Stand tall in front of a chair or step, take a big step forward and place your back foot on the chair or step.
• Bend your front knee and lower your body without leaning forward, keeping your back straight.

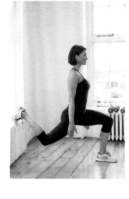

01

02 Suitcase swing
Butt, legs, core
• Grab your weights and stand tall with your feet hip width apart.
• Imagine your weights are suitcase handles.
• Lower into a squat, keeping your body weight in your heels and swinging your weights behind you.
• Push into your heels as you stand up tall.
• With straight arms, swing your weights above your head.
• Make sure your abs are tight and your core is engaged throughout.

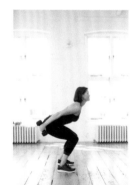
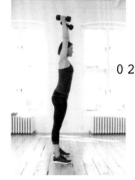

02

03 Full press up and kneeling press up
Chest, triceps, core, abs
• Assume the plank position.
• Gently lower your body towards the floor keeping your elbows pointing backwards.
• Keep your core engaged and your stomach tight – your body should be in a straight line from head to heels.
• As your body almost touches the floor push back up.
• Now come onto your knees and perform 3 kneeling push ups as in Week Two, Workout 2.

03

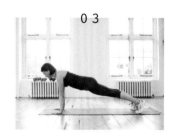
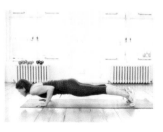
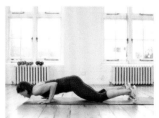

04 **Crouch jumping Jacks (as in Week One, Workout 2)**
Cardio, fat burn
- Stand tall with your feet together, heels off the floor on your tip toes.
- Lower your butt down to your heels and place your fingertips on the floor in front of you.
- Jump up and spread your arms and legs out to make an X shape.
- Land straight back into your crouch position and repeat.

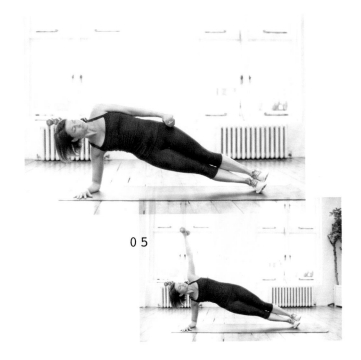

05 **Low side plank with arm raise (25 seconds each side)**
Waist, back, shoulder, core
- Lie down on your right side holding a weight in your left hand. Raise into a low side plank as we did in Week Three, Workout 1 (see page 229).
- Start with the weight at your left hip and, with a straight arm, raise it into a T position.
- Lower the weight back to your hip and repeat for 25 seconds.
- Swap sides and repeat.

06 **Egg roll to stand (as in Week Two, Workout 3, but finishing in a standing position)**
Cardio blast, fat burn, core, leg, shoulders
- Perform the exercise as for Week Two, but as you roll forward and swing your arms forward, use the momentum to come onto your feet, pushing into your heels and standing up tall.
- Bend your knees to sit back onto the floor and repeat.
- Too hard? Use your hands to give you a little push as you begin to stand up, or stay with the Week Two version.

To finish
5 minute stretch

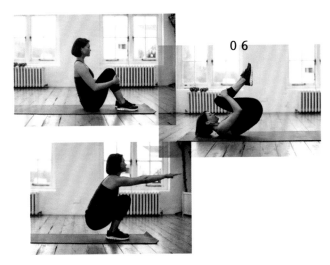

Week three

WORKOUT 3

3–5 minute warm up

01 **Skipping (as in Week One, Workout 1)**
Cardio
• Try to pick up the pace a little with smooth single jumps.

02 **360-degree lunge (front/side/back weighted)**
Inner, outer, front and back thigh, core
• This move brings together the forward, side and back lunges we have been doing in the first couple of weeks.
• Stand tall with your feet hip width apart and holding your weights by your sides.
• Perform a forward lunge and push back into the standing position.
• With the same leg, move into a side lunge, pushing back into the standing position.
• With the same leg, step back into a backward lunge.
• From the standing position, repeat with the other leg.

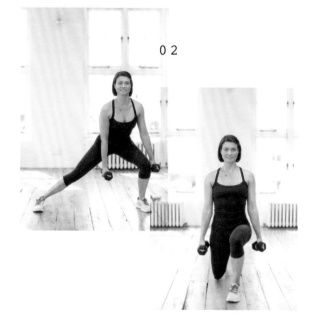

03 **Woodchop (25 seconds each side)**
Back, thighs, shoulders, core, waist
• Stand tall, with your feet shoulder width apart, holding a single weight with both hands.
• Squat down, touching the weight on your left foot.
• Stand back up whilst raising the weight above your right shoulder.
• Twist from left to right, bringing your left heel off the ground as you reach up.
• Imagine you are chopping down a tree.
• Repeat, alternating from your right foot to your left shoulder.

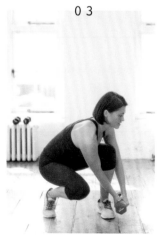

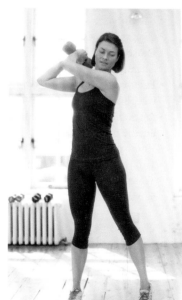

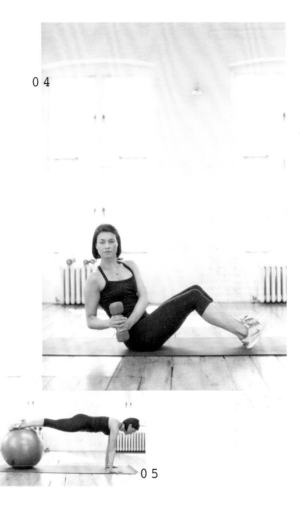

04 **Russian twists**
Waist, back, core
- Sit on the floor with your feet together, heels on the floor and knees bent.
- Hold a weight with both hands slightly in front of your body.
- Lean back a few inches (slightly) and engage your abs.
- Twist so the weight is moving from one side to another.
- Picture yourself rowing down the Amazon in a canoe.

05 **High plank on Swiss ball**
Core, shoulders, abs
- Get onto all fours with a Swiss ball at your feet.
- One leg at a time, place your feet and shins on the Swiss ball.
- Assume the high plank position with both feet and shins steadily on the Swiss ball.
- Be sure to engage your core and tense those abs to keep a nice straight line from your head all the way down to your heels.

06 **Low side plank (25 seconds per side)**
Waist, core
- Lie on your side.
- Place your right elbow directly beneath your shoulder.
- Raise your hips off the ground so your body is in a straight line from head to heels.
- Lift your left arm up into a T shape then lower, wrapping it under your body.
- After 20 seconds, gently lower, turnover and repeat on the other side.

To finish
5 minute stretch

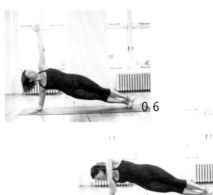

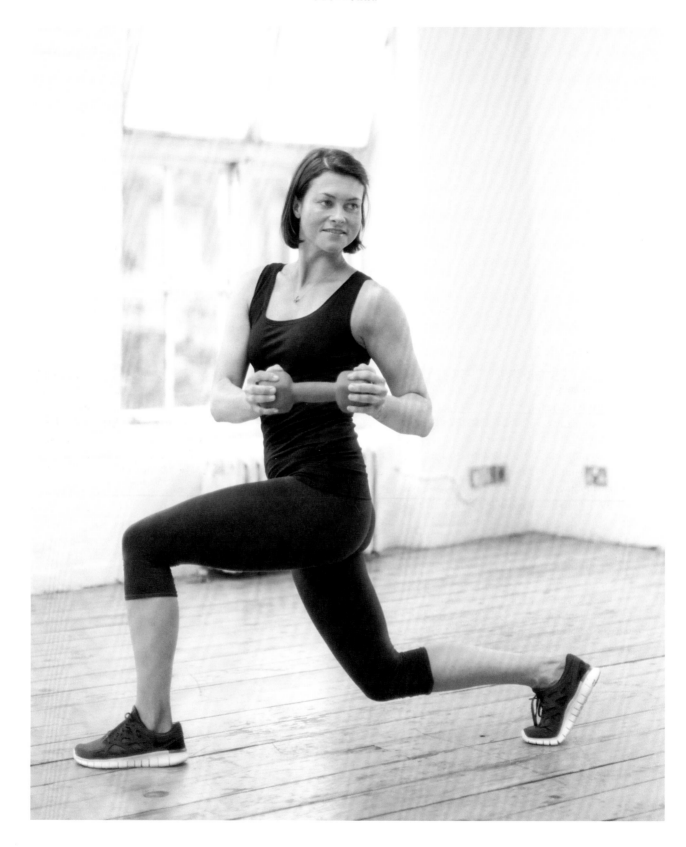

WEEK FOUR

get hooked

Timing

60 seconds on each exercise

0 seconds between exercises

Repeat circuit 3 times

30 seconds rest between each circuit

Tips for the week ahead

Workout 1

Burpees (page 236) are the king of cardio and the more burpees you do, the quicker you'll see results. Turn that hate into love and watch the fat melt off.

Your glute (butt) muscle is the biggest in your body. The more muscle you have, the more calories your body burns, even when resting. Fire up your glutes and make that muscle burn today.

As the saying goes 'Fail to prepare, prepare to fail', so get your healthy food ready the night before and have your healthy snacks always on hand.

Workout 2

Triceps – banish those bingo wings! Get the biggest muscle in your arm burning for that lean and toned look.

If you still look cute at the end of your workout, then you didn't train hard enough. Sweat and red faces are all good when it comes to exercising!

When it gets tough, smile to yourself and be content. You are doing a wonderful thing for your body right now!

Any exercise where you have weights above your head is amazing for strengthening your abs.

The crazy monkey (page 239) is a great core exercise, so make sure your core is tight and engaged throughout.

Workout 3

You should be feeling fit and strong, well done for getting this far. There's no rest in between each exercise – feel the burn and don't give up. The wonderful feeling of 'I did it!' at the end of this workout will be a great reward for all your effort.

Week four

WORKOUT 1

3–5 minute warm up

01 **Burpee**
Cardio, fat burn, full body
- Assume the high plank position (see Week One, Workout 3).
- Engage your core and jump your knees towards your chest as in a squat thrust.
- Smoothly transfer your weight to your legs, keeping your feet beneath your knees.
- From this crouching position jump up reaching up with your hands.

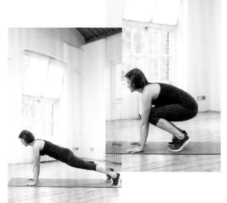
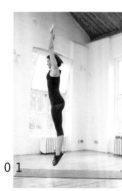

01

02 **Bridge with single leg raise**
Butt, back, thighs, core
- Lie on your back with your knees bent and feet hip width apart.
- Engage your stomach muscles and 'zip up' your pelvic floor. Push your heels into the floor to raise your hips.
- Hold this position and raise one leg off the ground so your knee is above your hip.
- Return your leg to the floor and then repeat the raise with the other leg. Try to keep your hips level.

02

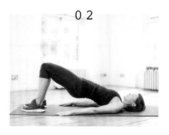
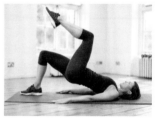

03 **Curtsy to knee raise with shoulder press**
(30 seconds per leg)
Butt, thighs, shoulders, balance, core
- Stand tall with your feet hip width apart and weights by your side.
- Step back with your right foot so it goes behind and outside the line of your left foot.
- Keeping your back straight, bend both legs so your front knee is at 90 degrees and you look as if you are curtsying. Touch the weights on the floor either side of your front foot and in line with your shoulders.
- Push back up and bring your knee to your chest.
- Raise the weights above your head.
- Repeat with the other leg.

03

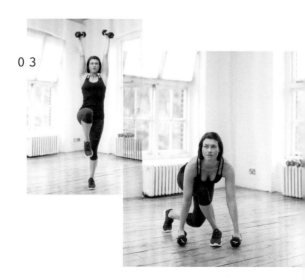

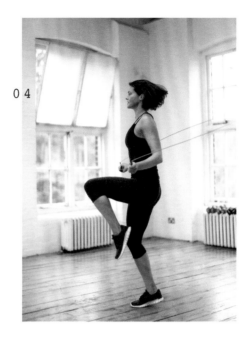

04 **Skipping**
Cardio, fat burn
- Our old favourite (see Week One, Workout 1). If you feel ready to step it up, start running on the spot while skipping.
- Drive those knees high as if you were sprinting.

05 **Jack-knife on Swiss ball**
Abs, shoulders, balance, core
- Get into a high plank position with your feet and shins on a Swiss ball (see Week Three, Workout 3).
- Engage your core and tense your abs to keep you nice and straight.
- Bring your knees up to your chest, rolling the ball under your shins and feet as you go.
- Keep your back straight and your shoulders over your hands.

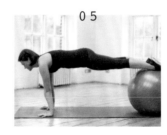
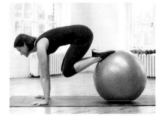

06 **Flies on Swiss ball**
Cardio blast, fat burn, core, leg, shoulders
- Grab your weights and sit on a Swiss ball.
- Walk your feet forward until just your head and upper back are on the ball.
- Raise the weights up with your arms in line with your shoulders.
- Engage your core and legs to keep stability on the ball.
- With palms facing each other and your arms slightly bent, lower the weights until your elbows are in line with your body.
- Raise back up to the starting position and repeat. Keep your hips lifted throughout and feel the burn.

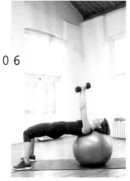
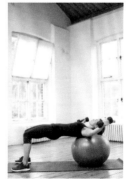

To finish
5 minute stretch

Week four

WORKOUT 2

3–5 minute warm up

01 Plié squat with high pull
Inner thighs, butt, upper back, core
- Grab your weights and stand with your feet wider than shoulder width apart with your toes and knees pointing outward – remember second position, ballet dancers.
- Hold the weights straight down in front of you, palms facing towards you.
- Keeping your back straight, squat down, making sure your knees stay in line with your toes.
- As you stand up, raise your elbows high to bring the weights under your chin.
- Keeping your shoulders relaxed, squeeze your shoulder blades together.
- Lower your arms and sit straight back into your plié squat.

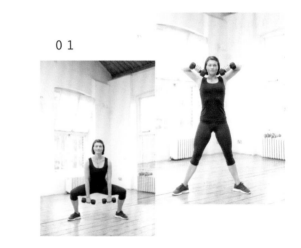

02 Single arm row to extension (T raise) (30 seconds per side)
Butt, back, thighs, core
- Stand tall with your feet shoulder width apart and a weight in your right hand.
- Take a lunge to your left. Place your left arm on your left thigh for support and hold.
- Start with the weight on the floor and keeping your arm close to your body lift the weight.
- When your arm is in line with your body twist, extend your arm and raise the weight above you, looking up to your raised hand.
- Slowly return to the start position, repeat for 30 seconds and swap sides.

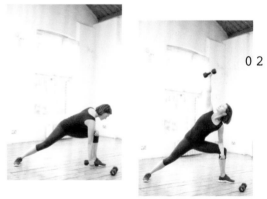

03 Running on the spot with weights above your head
Cardio, legs, shoulders, core
- Grab your weights and hold them straight above your head. Tighten and engage your core.
- Run on the spot by bringing your knees up to your chest.

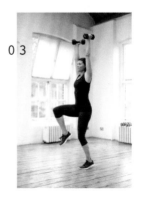

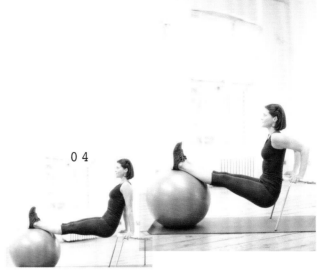

04 **Tricep dips**
Triceps, core, balance
- Sit on the edge of a chair with your hands on the chair, fingers facing forward.
- Either keep your legs straight out in front of you or rest them on a Swiss ball.
- Taking your weight in your arms, lower your body towards the floor, keeping your back close to the chair.
- Bend your elbows to 90 degrees and push back up.
- Your triceps will burn, but don't forget that your core is always working.

05 **Crazy monkey (handstand leg flicks)**
Shoulders, back, abs, core, legs
- Place your hands on the floor under your shoulders.
- Bend your knees and stick your butt in the air.
- Keep your weight over your hands and jump your feet off the floor trying to kick your butt with your heels.
- Go as high as you can – think handstand and one day you might get there – have fun!

06 **Lunge with weighted rotation**
Thighs, butt, waist, core
- Grab one weight and hold it in both hands close to your chest.
- Step forward into a lunge and, as you do this, rotate your body so it is facing over your front leg.
- Keep your back straight and core strong.
- Push back to the start position and repeat on the other side.

To finish
5 minute stretch

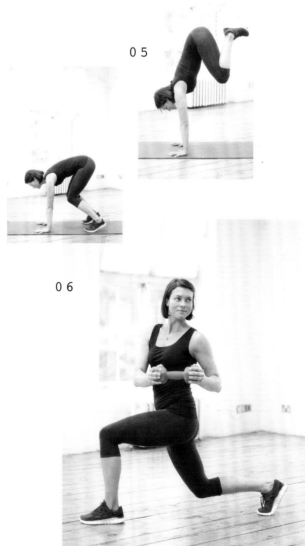

Week four

WORKOUT 3

3–5 minute warm up

01 **Jumping scissor lunges**
Cardio blast, fat burn, legs, butt
- Step forward into a lunge position but only drop half as deep into the lunge.
- Quickly jump up and switch legs mid-air, landing softly on opposite legs.
- Keep your back straight.
- This move should be fast and dynamic.

02 **Balancing tricep kickbacks (30 seconds on each side)**
Triceps, butt, legs, core
- Grab your weights and stand with your feet hip width apart.
- Balance on one foot and bend forward from the hips.
- Extend your raised leg behind you, letting it bend slightly.
- Keep your elbows close to your sides and straighten your arms, lifting the weights up in line with your sides. Focus on a spot in front of you to maintain your balance.

03 **Squatting wall sit**
Butt, thighs, shoulders, arms
- Get into a squat position, pressing your lower back and shoulders flat against the wall.
- Make sure your butt is in line with your knees and your thighs are parallel to the floor. Keep your knees over your ankles.
- Hold your squat and extend your arms straight out in front of you.
- Rotate your arms from the 'thumbs up' position to the 'thumbs down' position for a full 60 seconds.

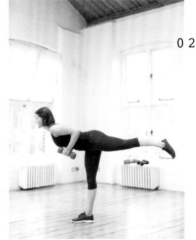
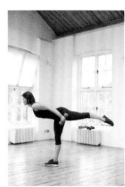

02

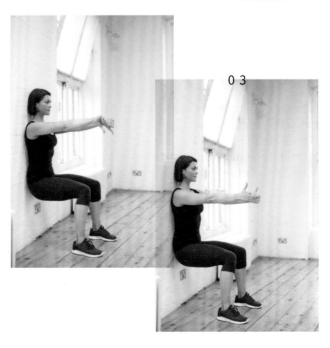

03

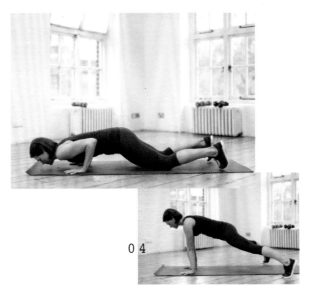

04 **Straddle jump with kneeling press up**
Cardio, fat burn, chest, triceps, abs
- Get into the high plank position (see Week One, Workout 1).
- Keep your core engaged and your stomach tight – your body should be in a straight line from head to heels.
- Jump your feet wide to a straddle then back to the start.
- Place your knees on the floor and do a kneeling press up.
- Repeat in this pattern.

05 **Mountain climbers**
Cardio, fat burn, shoulders, abs, legs
- Start in the high plank position (see Week One, Workout 1).
- Bring one knee into your chest.
- Quickly swap legs and bring the other knee to your chest.
- Keep changing legs as fast as you can while maintaining the plank position.

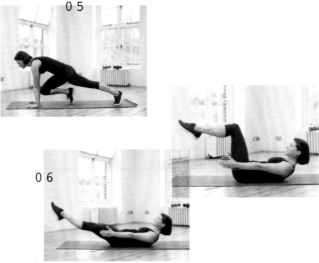

06 **Saucer**
Abs, thighs
- Lie on your back with your arms by your sides.
- Bring your legs into a table top position – knees over hips and ankles in line with knees.
- Engage your core and gently press your lower back into the floor.
- Lift your head, chest and arms off the floor. Extend your legs in front of you at 45 degrees. Hold for 60 seconds.
- If this is too much, bring your legs back into the start position and raise your arms and body only.

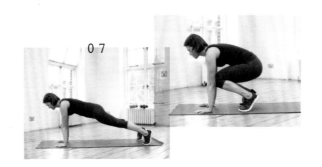

07 **Squat thrust**
Abs, thighs
- Start in a high plank position (see Week One, Workout 1).
- Jump your feet as close to your hands as you can.
- Then jump both feet back into a high plank. Repeat.

To finish
5 minute stretch

Don't have time?

TIME TO TABATA!

Tabata training is seriously effective at burning fat and improving cardio. It's a workout that is super short (4 minutes in total) and done with super high intensity.

This training technique was created by Izumi Tabata, a Japanese scientist, in the early 1990s after carrying out tests on two groups of athletes. The first undertook moderate intensity workouts, lasting an hour, and the second were trained to do high intensity interval training (HIIT) workouts lasting only 4 minutes: 20 seconds of all-out effort followed by a 10-second rest, repeated eight times. The results showed that HIIT increased the aerobic and basal metabolic rate of anyone who used it.

HIIT or Tabata training fires up your metabolism during the workout and keeps it fired up long after you have finished, creating the after-burn effect. So you continue to burn calories long after your workout has finished, which increases your metabolism. Having a high metabolism will help you burn fat. The benefits for this high intensity training are clear, but it should be used in addition to, not as a replacement for, other types of training. It's all about getting a balance and keeping it varied.

Tabata is for people who have successfully made it through my four week workout programme (pages 211–241). Because of its high intensity, Tabata could be dangerous for anyone at risk from strokes and heart attacks. If you have high blood pressure, consult with your doctor before performing Tabata or HIIT exercises.

Now to give it a go. First download the Tabata or Gymboss interval timer app to help you keep to your 4-minute workout. Remember it's 20 seconds of all your effort and a 10-second rest. Make sure you have warmed up properly before you start a Tabata workout.

The aim is to give it everything you have – 20 seconds to smash it! You do eight rounds in total. Each exercise lasts for 20 seconds with 10 seconds rest. Do all four exercises, one after the other, then repeat. Done!

Tabata Workout 1
• 20 seconds of Burpees (page 236)
10 second rest
• 20 seconds of Mountain climbers (page 241)
10 second rest
• 20 seconds of Fast feet with sprinter's arms (page 223)
10 second rest
• 20 seconds of Press-ups (page 230)
Repeat

Tabata Workout 2
• 20 seconds of Squat thrusts (page 228)
10 second rest
• 20 seconds of Crouch jumping jacks (page 215)
10 second rest
• 20 seconds of Caterpillar walkouts (page 207)
10 second rest
• 20 seconds of Egg rolls to stand (page 231)
Repeat

CONCLUSION

After all is said and done, after all the kids are ready for school with bags packed and out the door, after all those early starts getting to work, cold and dark in the middle of a frosty winter's morning, after all those late nights, sitting at the computer writing into the small hours of the morning, it's easy to forget the love that we need to give to ourselves.

There is a certain love and care that we should all give ourselves daily and there are many trappings that we can fall into in modern life, but there is a way to make things easier and more enjoyable, to be able to live life with a little more joy and contentment. This book has been, for the three of us, a way of putting in one place all the things we share with each other. It's a book to remind ourselves of how to hold onto that joy and stay with the contentment, we all need reminding of how to do that sometimes.

In some moments, life can get a little unmanageable and we can start to slip. It's best to just draw a line under that moment and start again, without any judgment and without giving yourself a hard time.

We are all constantly seeking and looking to continuously learn and grow, yet we still mess up, we still make mistakes. We are far from perfect, but it's important to each of us to maintain a sense of self love and self awareness and to carry on trying our best.

On the pages in this book, we don't propose a hardcore regime – it's a book that you can pull off the shelf time and time again to gain inspiration and get back on track, at any time of year.

It's been a huge privilege, lots of hard work and endless laughs for us to write this book. We hope you have as much fun with it as we have had writing it.

With love from Sadie, Holly and Amber xxx

KNOWLEDGE IS POWER

BE PREPARED

Relying solely on your willpower is risky, and it's not likely to work. It's better to be prepared instead. If you go too long without food, your blood sugar levels will drop and that's when you'll find yourself tempted by a quick fix – usually high sugar and trans fats snacks. You can try to avoid this by not having anything unhealthy in the house in the first place, and making sure you always carry a healthy snack with you for when you're out and about.

Read your labels

Get wise to packaging. You will be surprised by what's actually in so-called 'natural', 'healthy', 'organic', 'fresh', 'low fat' food products. Lots of these cleverly marketed packaged foods and snacks are not so good for you at all – so read labels carefully. Foods are often filled with stabilisers, emulsifiers, E-numbers, high-fructose sweeteners, corn syrup and other equally nasty ingredients. 'Low fat' products are some of the worst – when taking out the fats, sugar is often added to combat the loss of flavour, which makes it even worse for you. Good fats are essential and not to be avoided. It's important to understand the difference between good and bad fats (see page 247). Understanding labels is key to making sure you are buying and eating the best possible health giving foods.

Sugar

Sugar is a drug – it's addictive!

Apart from being a highly toxic and harmful substance, sugar is responsible, at least in part, for the following:
• Weight gain/obesity
• Tooth decay and gum disease
• Diabetes
• Mood swings
• Depression
• Anxiety
• Hormonal imbalances
• Depletion of nutrients from deep within the body
• Premature ageing of the body and skin
• Dullness and congestion within the skin
• Low energy levels

Daily consumption of sugar produces a continuously alkaline over acid condition. Consequently, minerals are required from deep within the body tissues, such as bones and teeth, in order to buffer the acidic environment and rectify the imbalance. So much calcium is taken from the bones and teeth that decay and general weakening begin. Consuming refined sugars eventually affects the whole body.

On top of that, a high sugar diet stops Leptin, the hormone that inhibits hunger when you are full, from working properly, so when we consume sugar we have a big tendency to over-eat.

Somehow we have to find a way of including treats and a little sweetness in our lives without doing the damage. We can achieve this by finding delicious, natural, health giving alternatives. Raw honey, pure Maple syrup, raw chocolate and fruit are great sugar alternatives that provide complex sugars, nourishment and essential micro nutrients to the body without depleting its own resources – and they taste amazing.

Water

Water is essential to a healthy mind, body and soul. Our bodies are over 60% water.

We need water in order to think clearly and flush the build up of toxins from within the body. Our brains are over 70% water and require a daily dose of pure clean water from foods, herbal teas and drinking water in order to function well and think clearly. The signs of dehydration are constipation, headaches, tiredness, and the feeling of hunger. Often when you think you're hungry, your body is actually trying to tell you that it's dehydrated. It's important to drink either filtered water or pure spring or mineral water to recieve the best benefits without any of the chemicals or additives in straight tap water. However, bottled mineral water is often stored in plastic bottles that contain BPA (Bisphenol A) which is an accumulative chemical that has been found to drastically increase the levels of oestrogen within the body, regardless of whether you are female or male. In males, this can cause prostate cancer and lowered sperm count. In females, it can cause breast cancer. In children and infants, BPA has been shown to promote hyperactivity. In addition, plastic bottles are insanely bad for the environment. A great way around this is to use BPA-free plastic, metal or glass bottles, that you can use again and again, by filling up with filtered water or spring water. This is not only cheaper, but its better for the environment and for your body.

Fruit and vegetables

In the past, most produce was left to fully mature before being harvested and used within a short distance of its source. Nowadays most commercially produced grains, fruits and some vegetables are harvested before they are fully ripened, which inevitably means reduced nourishment. For example, produce picked early doesn't develop as many sunlight related nutrients such as anthocyanins and polyphenols, compounds that give fruit their colour and flavour and which protect against DNA damage, brain cell deterioration and cancer. The best way around this is to grow and/or source fruits and vegetables that are as local and seasonal as possible. This kind of produce is most often found in farmers markets, in certain 'What's in season' sections in the super market, or on your neighbour's apple tree!

Grains, nuts and seeds – to soak or not to soak

Grains, nuts, legumes and seeds are rich in enzymes. However, unsoaked or sprouted, they also contain enzyme inhibitors such as phytic acid, a substance present in the bran of all grains, nuts and seeds. It inhibits the absorbtion of calcium, magnesium, iron, copper and zinc, and makes them hard to digest. Sprouting or soaking neutralises the enzyme inhibitors present in all grains nuts and seeds, making them easy to digest and much more nutritious – this has always been done in traditional cultures. By soaking and/or sprouting, you are in effect mimicking the process of germination. This increases the enzyme activity by as much as six times, making them much more nutritionally valuable. I always soak my grains, nuts and seeds. Homemade sprouts are fun to make and so delicious added to salads and sandwiches.

Detox your pantry

It's a great idea to detox your pantry. Clear out anything that doesn't support your health. That way, you won't be tempted by toxic snacks when you're hungry or tired. Having only delicious and health-giving ingredients in your fridge and pantry will help you to stay on your path of eating nourishing, wonderful food.

Caffeine

Caffeine is a stimulant. An excess (more than two cups a day) can place a huge amount of stress on the adrenal glands, causing your body to produce excess amounts of the hormones adrenaline and cortisol. These hormones help the body respond to stress and, when there is too much of it flooding your system, it will make the body store fat. Too much caffeine can also contribute to cellulite, as it impedes the circulation of nutrients to the skin, also depleting the skin of important nutrients like calcium and vitamin B. As caffeine is a diuretic, it can make you dehydrated and contribute to water retention in your body. It's not all bad though; having one (no more than one) cup of good-quality organic coffee a day can give the body antioxidants and help aid digestion. The same goes for green tea. As it contains less caffeine than coffee, you can drink more of it, and it is much higher in the lovely antioxidants that are so good for the body. Avoid decaffeinated drinks completely, as they have been highly processed.

Portion tip

So you're being super-healthy and feeling great for it, but make sure you're aware of portion sizes – use your hand as guide.

Palm = Proteins: this will include fish, poultry, legumes (beans, etc.), tofu and tempeh.

Fist = Carbohydrate: whole grains and rice etc.

Hand = Vegetables: a spread hand is a good portion (the greener the better)

Thumb = Fats: good, healthy fats.

LIFESTYLE

If you want to achieve a healthier lifestyle in a realistic way, remember the ratio of 90:10. If you follow your healthy approach 90 per cent of the time, you can allow yourself the remaining 10 per cent to relax and enjoy yourself. This means you can still enjoy treats, but try to make sure they stay in the 10 per cent and don't become habit. You should never just write a day off and think that, because you have slipped up, you might as well let your healthy approach go. Life is constantly moving forward, so leave your moment of weakness behind and move forward.

Say no to the ready-meal

Processed food is the enemy, as it has been altered from its natural state. Foods that were once nutritious have been so highly processed that they then have to have an array of different artificial ingredients added back into them to make them taste good. Bulking agents and fillers mean that processed food is cheaper to buy and added preservatives mean that it will last a long time sitting on the supermarket shelf.

They then no longer contain any of the good micronutrients and enzymes our bodies need. Although these convenience foods can seem tempting, there are so many other ways that are quick, simple, cheap and delicious to feed yourself and/or your family. Check out the recipes in this book it see how easy it is to make healthy delicious fast food.

No fad diets

Most people (including all three of us) have tried strict diets and crazy hardcore exercise plans… do they work? Yes, they can do initially. But are they sustainable? No! Does the weight you lose always come back? Yes! Are you enjoying the exercise? No. Is it healthy? No.

Trying to follow a strict diet or full-on training regime can be super tough. You go for it 100% with the best intentions. You start to see results and you think that there is no stopping you… but life gets in the way. You have a stressful day, the kids are sick, you're behind with a major deadline at work and you're exhausted, so you skip your gym session. You throw a pizza in the oven and, as you've blown the diet anyway, you down half bottle of wine, too. In one quick moment your great routine has fallen apart. Then you spend the rest of the night feeling guilty. You feel like all the hard work you have put in over the last few weeks is for nothing, and you slip back into your old routine.

Not only does your body start to yo-yo in weight, but also it puts a huge amount of stress on your body's metabolism. Find your balance. Small changes make a big difference, don't try and do it all at once.

Chewing

Taking your time to chew your food is seriously important. Chewing makes saliva that breaks down your food, so it can be digested properly. If you eat too fast and swallow lumps of un-chewed food, it will sit in your stomach undigested for a long time, causing bloating and wind. If you eat a nutritious meal and don't chew it properly, a lot of the vitamins and minerals contained in the food won't be released. Take your time over every meal and chew each mouthful at least 20 times. For a flatter, happier tummy, it's time to chew.

Alcohol

Alcohol is a popular way to cope with stress. It's relaxing, it's legal, and it's everywhere. But alcohol is the simplest and most fattening sugar of them all. Full of empty calories, it's super toxic and causes damage to almost every part of the body, from the internal organs to the skin. Drinking alcohol decreases your muscle mass, which will leave your body soft and out of shape. Being aware of the side effects of alcohol is important, so it doesn't become the go-to stress relief at the end of each day.

Moderation is key, so the occasional glass of red wine or a cooling G&T is fine. It's not about denying yourself the ritual or pleasure, it's about replacing it with delicious and health-giving alternatives.

pH levels

The aim is to keep acid low. Your body is constantly working to keep your pH levels in balance and we can help it along by eating the right things. Acid-forming foods like refined sugars, meat, wheat and processed foods aren't good for the body. An acid body is like magnet for disease, sickness, cancer and aging. Alkaline foods keep your body healthy and functioning properly. High alkaline foods include most vegetables, wheatgrass, almonds, some fruits, and seeds.

Stop counting calories

We've got to step away from the idea that all calories are created equal. They are not. Here's a great example: take one Mars bar and one and a half avocados; they have roughly the same number of calories. However, the way in which your body processes these two foods couldn't be more different. When you consume the Mars bar, your body effectively recognises it as poison – your built-in alarm systems kick into gear and a chemical process happens which takes the poisons out of your blood stream and into your fat cells. On the other hand, when you eat an avocado, your body recognises it as a nourishing food source. It is able to absorb all those wonderful calories and turn them into cellular building blocks and life-giving energy for your body to function properly. It then pushes anything it doesn't require through the digestive system and out the other end.

Mars bars = toxins = fat = cravings = moodiness.

Avocado = energy = nourishment = satisfaction = happiness

It's not about counting calories, but making sure the calories you are eating are the good ones.

FATS
The Good, the Bad & the Ugly

The Human brain is about 60% fat (dry weight). Every membrane of every cell and every organelle inside of cells are made of fats. Many hormones, neurotransmitters and other active substances in the body are made of fats. Fats are extremely important in our diet. The big question is: which fats?

Let us first tell you about margarines, butter replacements, 'spreadable' vegetable oils, shortenings and many other artificial fats. They are hydrogenated to increase their shelf life and to make them the right consistency. You can find hydrogenated oils in most processed foods, such as chocolates, ice cream, biscuits, cakes, breads, pastries, ready meals, crisps, etc. Hydrogenation is a process of adding hydrogen molecules to the chemical structure of oils under high pressure at a very high temperature (120°C

to 210°C or 240C to 410°C) in the presence of nickel, aluminium and sometimes other heavy metals. Remnants of these metals stay in the hydrogenated oils. Nickel and aluminium are both heavy metals, adding to the general toxic load which the body has to work hard to get rid of. Heavy metals, particularly aluminium, have been linked to many degenerative conditions, including Alzheimer's disease and dementia. But that is not the main problem with hydrogenated oils. Hydrogenation changes the chemical structure of the oils, producing a whole host of very harmful fats, more commonly known as 'trans fats'. Trans fatty acids are very similar in their structure to their natural counterparts, but they are somewhat back to front. Because of their similarity, they occupy the place of essential fats in the body while being unable to do their job, making cells in a way disabled. All organs and tissues in the body are affected. For example, transfats have great immune-suppressing ability, playing a detrimental role in many different functions of the immune system. They have been implicated in diabetes and neurological conditions, and they interfere with pregnancy, conception, the normal production of hormones... the list is long.

Fats are essential, but which ones should we consume, and how? Fatty acids keep our hair and skin glowing and support our brains and organs. Fats also help us to absorb fat-soluble vitamins that we want from the vegetables we eat. Essential Fatty acids are just that – essential!

• Fat enhances the flavor and texture of food.

• Fat provides us with fuel throughout the day.

• Fat boosts brain power.

The important thing to remember is that we should only consume fats that are in their natural state. without processing them. Oils must be cold pressed and raw. Eat fats as nature intended them and you will not go wrong.

For searing, browning & pan-frying (cold pressed and or raw)
• Safflower oil
• Sunflower oil
• Ghee
• Coconut oil
• Ground nut oil
• Goose fat/duck fat

Sautéing & oven baking
• Safflower oil
• Sunflower oil
• Ghee
• Coconut oil
• Ground nut oil
• Goose fat/duck fat
• Olive oil
• Rapeseed oil
• Grapeseed oil
• Sesame oil

Salad dressings, marinades, dips
• Walnut oil
• Pumpkin seed oil
• Avocado oil
• Flax seed oil
• Extra virgin olive oil
• Sesame seed oil
• Hazelnut oil
• Rapeseed oil

Oils for supplementation
• A good nut/ seed oil blend – 2:1 ratio of omega 3 to 6 fatty acids
• Cod liver oil
• Fish oil with a higher ratio of fatty acids EPA or DHA.

Love, Holly & Amber xx

NOURISH WEEK

The aim for this week is to nourish your body from inside out. To be gentle and kind to yourself, to take time out of your busy life to focus on you. The Nourish Week can be a warm up to the Cleanse & Tone Week (pages 250–251), giving you a 2-week programme, which we do ourselves, and it feels amazing. The idea of a Nourish Week is not to go on some crazy elimination diet where we end up feeling awful and have loads of withdrawal symptoms, but to simply really nourish your body so you feel energised, calm, replenished and recharged.
Love, Sadie xx

Monday	Morning: 6–10 Sun Salutations (pages 132–133) Evening: 5–10 minutes of Following the Breath (page 142)
Tuesday	A 20 minute mindful walk/jog, really being present in the moment
Wednesday	Morning: 6–10 Sun Salutations (pages 132–133) Evening: 5–10 minutes of Following the Breath (page 142)
Thursday	A 20 minute mindful walk/jog, really being present in the moment
Friday	Morning: 10 Sun Salutations (pages 132–133) Evening: 5–10 minutes of Following the Breath (page 142)
Saturday	A 20-minute mindful walk/jog, really being present in the moment
Sunday	Morning: 5–10 minutes of Following the Breath (page 142)

This eating plan can be adapted to meet certain dietary requirements. If you're vegetarian, swap the fish or chicken for a different veggie option in the mains section. If you don't eat grains or dairy, simply replace the milk or kefir in the smoothies with full-fat coconut milk or almond milk and use coconut cream or yoghurt for the granola or fruit salad. I am sure there will be meals where you will be either out or just fancy taking a break. If that's the case, just try to make wise decisions and avoid sugar and refined carbs. Remember, the more you nourish yourself, the less you will need the bad stuff.

Love, Amber xx

	Breakfast	Snack	Lunch	Snack	Dinner
Monday	Banana & Almond Smoothie (page 17)	A herbal tea and any snack from the list below	Nourish Bowl (page 66)	A herbal tea and any snack from the list below	Puy Lentils with Wilted Spinach (page 53) and a piece of pan–fried fish*
Tuesday	Avocado on rye toast or Cauliflower Toast (page 34)	A herbal tea and any snack from the list below	Nourish Bowl (page 66)	A herbal tea and any snack from the list below	Japanese Chicken (page 68) with Smashed Cucumber Salad (page 56) and quinoa or brown rice*
Wednesday	Som Tum Pollamai (page 47) with your favourite yoghurt	A herbal tea and any snack from the list below	Nourish Bowl (page 66)	A herbal tea and any snack from the list below	Spring Courgetti with Kale Pesto (page 80)*
Thursday	Blackberry, Rose & Raw Chocolate Smoothie (page 14)	A herbal tea and any snack from the list below	Nourish Bowl (page 66)	A herbal tea and any snack from the list below	My Mum's Veg Chilli (page 79)*
Friday	A smoothie of your choice (pages 14–17)	A herbal tea and any snack from the list below	Nourish Bowl (page 66)	A herbal tea and any snack from the list below	Lemon & Sumac Chicken (page 70) and Quinoa with a Rainbow of Jewels (page 62)*
Saturday	Poached Eggs with Cauliflower Toast (page 34)	A herbal tea and any snack from the list below	A soup of your choice (pages 50–52)	A herbal tea and any snack from the list below	Japanese Brown Rice Bowl and Kimchi (page 67) or Baked Pollock with Ginger (page 76)*
Sunday	Coconut & Banana Pancakes (page 33)	A herbal tea and any snack from the list below	Late lunch/early dinner: Mexican Feast (pages 72–73)		

Snacks

Choose from the following:
- A handful of soaked raw almonds
- 1 orange
- 2 Medjool dates
- 1 or 2 Spiced Chocolate & Sweet Potato Brownies (page 96), depending on size
- A few Coconut & Apricot Bliss Balls (page 91)
- A handful of blueberries

*You can follow any dinner with an optional dessert from the Sweet Tooth section (pages 83–103)

CLEANSE & TONE WEEK

The aim for this week is to cleanse the body from the inside and to really push and challenge your body from the outside. The Cleanse & Tone week is great to do if you really want to feel fab for an event, or a holiday or special occasion coming up. Pick a workout programme week that suits your level of fitness.

Love, Holly xx

Monday	• Warm up (pages 206–207) • Day 1 from programme of your choice (pages 211–241) • Stretches
Tuesday	• Warm up (pages 206–207) • 15 minutes skipping • One Tabata programme (page 242) • Stretches
Wednesday	• Warm up (pages 206–207) • Day 2 from programme of your choice (pages 211–241) • Stretches
Thursday	• 30-minute jog • Stretches
Friday	• Warm up (pages 206–207) • Day 3 from programme of your choice (pages 211–241) • Stretches
Saturday	• 30-minute jog • Stretches
Sunday	• Warm up (pages 206–207) • 15 minutes skipping • One Tabata programme (page 242) • Stretches

*This eating plan is a litte bit stricter than the Nourish week.
The best way to make it through each of these plans is to do a
little forward planning and get your self organised with at least
a day's worth of food ready to go in the fridge and pantry. Try
to go through this part of gathering, shopping and preparing
in a positive way. Don't think of it as chore, but as part of the
creative, learning and growing process we all have to go through
to love and nourish ourselves.*

Love, Amber xx

	Breakfast	*Snack*	*Lunch*	*Dinner*
Monday to Friday	A Green Juice (page 21) or a smoothie (pages 14–17) and/or Som Tum Pollamai (page 47) with yoghurt or A bowl of fresh fruit and a sprinkle of Grain-free Granola (page 40)	A herbal tea and any snack from the list below	A soup of your choice (pages 50–52) or a Nourish Bowl (page 66)	Choose from the Dinners listed in Nourish week (page 249), but try to avoid carbs and late-night eating
Saturday	Poached Eggs with Cauliflower Toast (page 34)	A herbal tea and any snack from the list below	A soup of your choice (pages 50–52) or a Nourish Bowl	Japanese Chicken (page 68) with Smashed Cucumber Salad (page 56) and a green leafy salad
Sunday	A Green Juice (page 21) or a smoothie (pages 14–17) and/or Som Tum Pollamai (page 47) with yoghurt or A bowl of fresh fruit and a sprinke of Grain-free Granola (page 40)	A herbal tea and any snack from the list below	Late lunch/early dinner: Mexican Feast (pages 72–73) or Lemon & Sumac Chicken (page 70) and Quinoa with a Rainbow of Jewels (page 62)	

Snacks
Choose from the following:
- A handful of soaked raw almonds
- 1 orange
- A handful of Kale Crisps (page 108)
- A few Coconut & Apricot Bliss Balls (page 91)
- A handful of blueberries
- Some raw vegetables with hummus

INDEX

ACKNOWLEDGEMENTS

Amber

There are a lot of people that I would like to show my thanks and love and gratitude to....

Firstly, I would like to thank my son: you are a constant source of love and inspiration and you keep me going. Thank you for all your patience and support, you really are the love of my life.

I would like to thank all the beautiful, talented, strong, incredible women in my life who have given me endless support and love and strength along the way to stay true to myself and keep going when things have not been easy: Vanessa Cooke, India Waters, Nandi Boyle, Beshlie Mckelvie, Nicola Guinness, Ali Allen – you have all made me who I am today and I love you all.

Thank you to Rosie Scott for her amazing support and guidance and for her endless encouragement in all areas of my life. You are amazing and I love you.

To Lucinda Carey: you are an amazing woman with so much to give. You have been such a huge support and I have so much love and respect for you and your beautiful children who I love and adore, thank you for your love along the way.

To Ieva Imsa and Ivor Guest, thank you for your support and strength,
you have been pillars in a sometimes rocky landscape. You are an inspiration and a joy to know.

Thank you to all the women in my family who have shared their love of food with me, midnight feasts and leisurely breakfasts, Sunday roasts and salads freshly picked from the garden. Vivien, Marion and Rachel, you rock – you're the best aunties anyone could ask for. Thank you Maida, I will never forget your crackling and your ginger nut biscuits and cups of steaming hot Milo on a cold winter's day.

Thank you Mum for growing the best garden full of the most amazing food that has spawned a life long obsession with food. I will always steal the first peaches, and fossick through the berry patch for the first berries, hope you don't mind!

I would also like to thank Sadie Frost and Holly Davidson for sharing this journey with me, for having the patience and love to keep going and plough through. You are both amazing and you are both an inspiration to me. Many more adventures to come.

Sadie

I would like to thank all my brothers and sisters and my Ma and Pa! My four beautiful children for keeping me young at heart.

Also thanks to all my gurus with whom I've studied yoga: Nadia Narain, Stewart Gilchrist, Bryony Bird, Luiz Veiga and the beautiful Hortense Suleyman. Hugh Poulton for showing me balance. Dan Burt for keeping me stretched and toned in Pilates.

Thanks to Yehudi Gordon for being there spiritually and with all the mind, body and soul I could have ever have needed. Nish Joshi for the acupuncture, healing and Zest and of course the lovely Chip and Heidi Somers who helped me through some of my most difficult times.

Also some of these people for showing me how it's done: Kate Moss, Jemima French, Emma Comley, Rose Ferguson and all my other spiritual fairies.

I would also like to thank all the fantastic teachers at Transcendental Meditation in London and Andy Puddicome from Head Space.

A big acknowledgement to the beautiful and spirited Zoe Grace and Jade Davidson from having the most lovely soul ever!

Holly

I would like to thank each and every one of my clients. You are all the reason why this book took flight. Thank you for your help, support, ideas and encouragement; you are all a daily inspiration to me. A special thanks to Sardia Khan and Sienna Guillroy.

Julie Lane, you are my guardian angel and words can't thank you enough for your help and time, and for taking me under your wing.

To Angelo Di Muro, thank you for setting me on the right tracks, for keeping your cool and for your fantastic organisation and planning.

I would like to thank all the mentors in my life. Their incredible knowledge and passion to teach has given me the hunger to learn more.

A special thanks to my first yoga teacher Gerry Ross, your smile and energy for life is contagious, and to Stewart Gilchrist, a magnificent guru who continues to challenge my body and mind.

Thank you, Dai Master Rafael Nieto, for making me strong and disciplined. And to all the senseis at Xen-Do who have taught me over the years. And Steve Harrison a great teacher, thank you for passing on your passion.

To my sister, Jade Davidson. I thank with all my heart, for your endless kindness, patience, wisdom and friendship. You are my shining star.

Thank you to all of my gorgeous family. Especially my niece and nephews Billy, Fin, Raff, Sean, Iris and Rudy for always making me smile.

Thank you to all the amazing friends I have around me. I love you all very dearly: Helen Bouillet , Jade Bevan, Natalie Ferstendik, Shelley Conn, Vicki Ballington, Bebhinn Gleeson, Triana Terry. And an extra big hug and love to Ania Sowiinski.

I'd like to send special thanks to my second family, The Baldwins – Tom, Rebecca, Frankie and Arthur – for your continuous support, love and friendship.

My NY boy, I want to thank you for your patience and support.

And of course a huge thanks to Sadie and Amber. You both have been pillars of strength and inspiration in my life. And to be able to have shared writing this book with you both has been such a wonderful journey. Thank you!

From the 3 of us

Firstly we would all like to thank Kyle, for her belief in this project, for her unwavering support and for cracking the whip when necessary – we would be nothing without you. Thank you for pulling this book together and giving us the support and guidance to shine. You have been utterly amazing, thank you!!!!

We would like to thank Heather Holden-Brown, our collective agent, for supporting us through this project and guiding us when we needed it. You have been a dream agent and we couldn't have got this far without you.

Thank you to David Loftus for bringing our vision to life, for your beautiful pictures and amazing eye. Thank you for all your hard work and support. You have given beauty and elegance to our project.

Thank you to Shiv, Fabiola, Jackie and Lilly for making us all gorgeous and beautiful and confident. You are all amazing talented ladies.

A special thank you goes out to Rukmini Iyer for your support and help in the kitchen.

Additional thanks to the following PR Agencies and suppliers for generously supplying the equipment and outfits used in this book:
Asquith London, Beshlie McKelvie (www.beshliemckelvie.com), Chinti and Parker, Didi Ilse Jewellery, Fabi-Atelier, Goodly PR, Karla Otto London, Isabel Marant, The Meditator, MIH Jeans, Nike, Zadig et Voltaire.

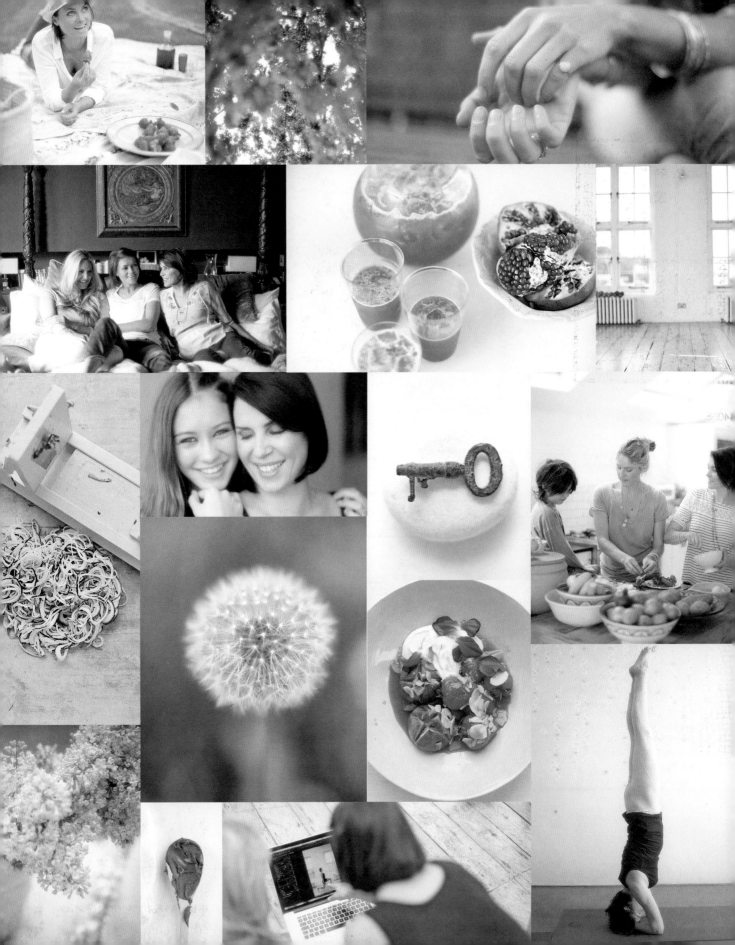